Health and Illness in a Changing Society

Health and illness are intensely personal matters. It seems self-evident that health is a basic necessity of the 'good life', though it is often taken for granted. Illness, on the other hand, challenges our sense of security and may introduce acute anxiety into our lives. At its extreme, illness threatens our very existence as individual beings. It is no wonder, therefore, that all societies mobilise cultural and material resources to deal with illness.

Yet health and illness are not simply human constants. For what appears, at one level, to be an intense individual experience, at another turns out to be of considerable social significance. The occurrence of illness varies by social position (e.g. class or gender) and the experience of ill health depends greatly on social context. *Health and Illness in a Changing Society* provides a sociological view of health and illness by considering key areas of current public and policy debate about health, and by critically analysing relevant academic research. The topics of the chapters have been selected to reflect the main areas of work in medical sociology. These are: health beliefs and behaviour, inequalities in health, the doctor–patient relationship, chronic illness and disability, death and dying, and the body and risk.

Health and Illness in a Changing Society provides a much-needed evaluative approach to new as well as established ideas in medical sociology.

Michael Bury is Professor of Sociology and Head of the Department of Social Policy and Social Science at Royal Holloway, University of London.

Health and Illness in a Changing Society

Michael Bury

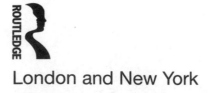

London and New York

First published 1997
by Routledge
11 New Fetter Lane, London EC4P 4EE

Simultaneously published in the USA and Canada
by Routledge
29 West 35th Street, New York, NY 10001

© 1997 Michael Bury

Typeset in Times by Routledge
Printed and bound in Great Britain by Biddles Ltd, Guildford and
King's Lynn

British Library Cataloguing in Publication Data
A catalogue record for this book is available from the British Library

Library of Congress Cataloguing in Publication Data
A catalogue record for this book has been requested

ISBN 0–415–11514–0 (hbk)
ISBN 0–415–11515–9 (pbk)

Contents

Illustrations

Acknowledgements

The essays that comprise the chapters of this book have arisen from research and teaching at Royal Holloway, University of London. Over the years I have benefited enormously from interactions and discussions with successive cohorts of masters students on the MSc programme in Medical Sociology taught at Royal Holloway. I have also been fortunate in recent years to work with colleagues who are experts in their fields of study. I am most grateful to Mary Ann Elston for her support and comments on early drafts of some of the chapters, and to Jonathan Gabe who gave me encouragement when I was flagging towards the end. He also read some of the chapters at that point. I am also grateful to Liz Young who read the chapter on death and dying. I have begged, borrowed and stolen ideas and insights from all three colleagues over the years, and from their comments now. I alone, of course, am responsible for what follows.

Introduction
Health, illness and sociology

Health and illness are intensely personal matters. It seems self-evident that health is a basic necessity of the 'good life'. As the refrain has it: 'if you have your health you have everything'. Illness, on the other hand, in all but its 'trivial' forms (and sometimes even then), challenges our sense of security and may introduce acute anxiety into our lives. At its extreme, illness threatens our very existence as individual beings; apart from taxes, death is the only certainty in life. It is no wonder, therefore, that all societies mobilise cultural and material resources to deal with illness. To be human is to be concerned with health and illness.

Yet health and illness are not simply human constants. For what appears, at one level, to be an intense individual experience, at another turns out to be of considerable social significance. Health and illness are social phenomena in at least two senses. First, few health disorders occur in a random fashion. Illness frequently varies by social group, whether this is couched in terms of class, gender, ethnicity or age. Health and illness are *socially patterned* and an individual's *social position* may have an important bearing on their experience (Macintyre 1986). The social patterning of illness is also *temporal* in character, whether this is conceived of in terms of its historical dimensions or the different stages of an individual's life course or biography (Blaxter 1992).

Second, health and illness are inevitably caught up in the social relationships that constitute our everyday lives and the wider society; at *micro* and *macro* levels. Health and illness are social phenomena because they inevitably have implications for the running of society. Political considerations come into play concerning the amount and distribution of economic resources that are given to promoting health or ameliorating illness. Not only that, but health and illness are part of the warp and weft of everyday reality. Our experiences of ill health immediately affect our relationships with others, as well as the carrying out of everyday tasks and the *presentation of self*. We cannot 'be ill' without simultaneously being aware of the need to account to others for our change in status.

This approach to the social character of health and illness, at once personal *and* social, puts it at the centre of the sociological imagination – that is, of the interaction between what Wright Mills called 'private troubles and public affairs' (Mills 1959). Yet for much of sociology's history (especially in Britain until the 1970s, and even afterwards) the field of health and illness, or the sub-discipline of medical sociology which has studied it, has not been seen as part of the mainstream. Though mental illness and psychiatry have long received attention in sociological writings in theories of deviance and social control, physical illness and 'ordinary' medical practice have, until recent times, been neglected by the parent discipline.

There are a number of possible reasons why this has occurred. Most important is that while sociologists have readily seen the social significance of subjects such as religion, education or the operation of labour markets, illness and medicine were not thought to have a direct bearing on the social or cultural fabric. With the exception of mental illness, most health disorders appeared to be 'natural' phenomena, treated by technical means, and thus in some way 'external' to the social structure. For a long time, social policy analysts treated the Health Service as if it was external to the economic system. Indeed, the health services were seen in opposition to the commercial sector; a cordoned-off 'socialised' area of modern society expressing collectivist values.

The world of professional medicine also appeared to be impenetrable to many sociologists, in comparison with the church or school. Only psychiatrists seemed fair game for sociological scrutiny, partly because in the 1960s and 1970s psychiatrists were themselves openly debating their differences and their undoubted chequered history in treating mental illness, a debate almost unheard of in other medical settings. And finally, medical sociological research appeared to many mainstream sociologists to be altogether too 'applied' and a-theoretical. This was a charge that some medical sociologists themselves accepted in an attempt to bring the 'parent' and specialist branches of the discipline closer together.

The neglect of health and illness as key sociological issues has changed dramatically over the last ten to fifteen years. Not only does medical sociology research continue to grow, in Britain and elsewhere, but health and illness are now considered as legitimate subjects in undergraduate sociology curricula as well as in professional training. Health and illness are also now recognised as being important subjects in the development of theoretical debates in sociology as well as substantive areas for empirical enquiry. Sociology textbooks now regularly feature health and illness as part of their mainstream fare, drawing attention to their importance in illustrating the 'sociological imagination'. Anthony Giddens, for example, uses health and illness in the introductory discussion to his textbook *Sociology*, stating that 'social factors have a profound effect on both the experience and occurrence of illness' (Giddens 1989: 9) and arguing that this illustrates the more general sociological proposition concerning the way in which 'our lives reflect the contexts of our social experience' (ibid.: 11).

In recent years, the theoretical importance of health and illness and of medical sociology has thus been more clearly recognised. While this book reflects this developing picture in its discussion of a number of key areas of medical sociology research, it does so within a framework emphasising change. Theoretical perspectives employed by medical sociologists in the 1970s are now being re-examined in the light of rapid changes in 'late modern' society, especially as they interact with health. Before providing an outline of the book's contents, it may be useful, therefore, to sketch in the main sociological perspectives that have been employed and shaped in medical sociology, and the ways in which these are now being refashioned.

PERSPECTIVES IN MEDICAL SOCIOLOGY

It is one of the contentions of this book that medical sociology relates to health and illness in two different ways. At one level, medical sociology tries to 'make sense of illness', to use Radley's phrase (Radley 1994), by applying its perspectives to the experience and social distribution of health disorders. At this level medical sociology often complements and sometimes challenges other disciplines that are concerned with health. Inevitably, medical sociology research touches on matters which are also of interest to clinical medicine, the bio-medical sciences, nursing, epidemiology and public health, and psychology. It is for this reason that, in practice, medical sociology research is often multidisciplinary in character. Many medical sociologists do not worry unduly about disciplinary labels.

On the other hand, the sociological study of health and illness, as has been indicated, opens an important window on more general social processes. The examination of the social patterning and experience of health and illness provides a mechanism for examining such matters as social inequalities, the nature of professional expertise and power and the links between self and society – themes that occur throughout this book. If medical sociology is to continue to make a distinctive contribution to the study of such matters, therefore, it also needs to retain a clear sense of its own disciplinary roots, even when working in a multidisciplinary setting. This is especially true when its perspectives are coming under pressure from the rapid transformation of social life. One of the few attempts to outline the conceptual foundations of medical sociology can be found in Gerhardt's book, *Ideas About Illness* (Gerhardt 1989). This provides a critical account of the sociological importance of health and illness, and informs the necessarily brief comments which follow. These act as a prelude to the contents of the chapters of the book.

The first sociological perspective which developed a distinctive analysis of health and illness was that of *functionalism*. This was concerned with the importance of health to the functioning of the social system as a whole. In the writings of Parsons (1951) and of his student Renée Fox (Parsons and Fox 1952), health was conceived of as one of the preconditions of social action. An optimum level of health in the population as a whole was seen as a prerequisite for the smooth functioning of modern society, based as it is on achievement and effective social organisation. Illness, both biological and 'socio-cultural' in origin, was conceptualised by Parsons as the inability of individuals to carry out their everyday tasks and social roles. This might be because of either the *incapacity* of the person to remain well in the face of disease or trauma, or a (partially motivated) tendency to fall ill in response to stress; in this latter instance illness was conceived of as a form of *deviance*. This tension in Parsons' work revealed the physical and psycho-social components that go to make up health and illness.

As far as responses to illness are concerned, Parsons followed through his functionalist perspective by regarding the patient's role as being a necessary means of channelling the threat involved in illness, both to the well-being of the individual and to society. The 'sick role' provided a means, for Parsons, through which the individual could temporarily 'deviate' and enter a dependent state, without threatening social cohesion at either the micro or macro level. The damage to social reciprocity brought about by illness could therefore be channelled into safe waters. The treatment of illness involved more than the relief of individual suffering. The growing influence of medicine demonstrated how science and rationality were becoming central to the construction of new forms of legitimate authority and social control in modern society.

This functionalist view of health, illness and medicine rested, arguably, on a rather simplistic view of social consensus, illustrated by the reciprocal if unequal doctor–patient relationship. If shared values could be maintained, this relationship (and, by implication, others in modern life) could proceed with relative smoothness, even in the face of inequality. However, many sociologists found it difficult to adhere to this generally positive view of modern social life, and to the functionalists' view that they could provide a comprehensive and scientific account of its workings. Parsons' work has probably been most influential as a foil for the development of alternative views that have been fashioned by subsequent generations of sociologists.

One of the main criticisms levelled against Parsons has been his apparent lack of attention to social change and to social conflict. Though some sociologists have argued that Parsons was concerned with system stability *in a period of rapid social change* (Holton and Turner 1986: 15), the absence of any serious discussion of change or conflict in Parsons' formulations of the sick role and the doctor's role, for example, is evident. During the 1960s and especially in the 1970s, a strong *conflict* perspective developed in reaction to this view, and became particularly influential in medical sociology.

The conflict perspective emphasised that, despite the contention that (capitalist) society had a stake in recognising and promoting positive health, a great deal of ill health went unrecognised. Surveys such as Wadsworth's (Wadsworth *et al.* 1971) showed that doctors dealt with only a small fraction of illness. Much illness went officially unrecognised and therefore untreated. Other empirical work also demonstrated that even severe symptoms did not necessarily lead to a positive social response or to medical treatment. Moreover, sociologists were also 'rediscovering' the presence of poverty in modern American and European contexts, and were showing how this was a powerful determinant of levels of morbidity (illness) and mortality (death). Thus social divisions and conflict were seen to be behind observed patterns of illness; health and illness were not just biological events or the result of ill-specified forms of social strain (as they had been in Parsons' formulation) but *socially created* through deprivation and social environmental breakdown (Gerhardt 1989: 267).

Conflict was also seen to be at the root of the doctor–patient relationship. Where Parsons had seen reciprocity and a functional handling of illness as deviance, writers such as Freidson (1970a) struck a very different note. Professional authority, legitimate and progressive for Parsons, was now seen as inherently damaging. For Freidson, the rational medical model was a means of exerting *medical dominance* over the patient and excluding the *lay construction* of illness from the clinical encounter. In this account, patients were preoccupied by their subjective experience of illness while doctors were preoccupied with disease. It was the doctors' 'definition of the situation' that prevailed. This approach to medical power formed part of a general sociological critique and a more negative view of professional power in modern societies.

Though the conflict perspective offered (and still offers) many medical sociologists a 'critical' alternative to the somewhat 'medico centric' approach to health and illness of functionalist sociology, there were a number of difficulties with its formulation. The most important of these, from the point of view of the current discussion, was that, despite charges that modern medical power was leading to 'medical imperialism' and the 'medicalisation of everyday life' (Zola 1972), much empirical research failed to show that these processes were strongly in evidence. In fact, lay people appeared to be far more 'active' in their handling of illness and medicine than conflict theory suggested (Dingwall 1976). Moreover, a 'medical dominance' form of reasoning also set up a tension, creating a 'no win' situation for medicine; the more it took patients' subjective views into account, the more it could be accused of incorporating ever increasing aspects of the patient's 'life world' into the medical orbit. In either case, medicine was portrayed as the culprit and sociology the innocent critic (Strong 1979a).

Somewhat disconcertingly, studies of patient views also tended to show consistently high levels of 'expressed satisfaction' with modern health care, and a persistent deference to doctors rather than hostility or conflict (Cartwright 1967; Cartwright and Anderson 1981). Though the importance of inequality in the occurrence of illness and in the use of services was widely promulgated by medical sociologists, much of the treatment of illness in the public view seemed to be associated with social progress. Indeed, overall health was improving in modern societies; with some exceptions in particular age groups, survival into old age was becoming the norm, and many forms of life-threatening illness were in decline. The depiction of the changing pattern of illness as the result of 'diseases of civilization' (Powles 1972) seemed to be at odds with the 'rediscovery of poverty' arguments being advanced in conflict-oriented and Marxian-influenced sociological writings.

An alternative approach, based on an *interactionist* perspective, developed alongside conflict theory, partly to tackle some of these weaknesses. Interactionist theory emphasised *negotiation* in both the occurrence and social responses to illness. In illness occurrence, a negotiated element was seen as central to the detection and naming of symptoms. In chronic disorders in particular, a series of exchanges were seen to take place between the individual and others as the 'negotiated reality' of the disorder unfolded. Chronic illness, entailing a long-term threat to self and identity, had to be negotiated with others in the attempt to maintain a sense of normality (Gerhardt 1989: 159). In an interactionist perspective, people did not so much 'fall ill' as 'become ill', with the outcome being contingent on a series of social exchanges. Interactionist theory emphasised the significance and meaning of behaviour rather than its causation (Burns 1992: 12).

By the same token, responses to illness, including those in professional–client relationships, could be characterised as a process of interaction, involving negotiation. In the functionalist perspective, clinical encounters were seen as a matter of compliance and reciprocity, and in the conflict view, as fraught by incipient breakdown. *Both* of these elements were seen to be potentialities in the interactionist perspective, as part of a *negotiated order*, whether in a hospital or clinic setting or in routine decision-making about treatment regimens.

The changing nature of illness over time also emerged as important in the negotiation perspective, with the response of lay people to managing the long-term effects of treatment being seen as equally important to the experience of symptoms. Agreements about the nature of the illness and its treatment, reached through negotiation whether in professional or lay circles, were seen to be influenced by the social context as the *trajectory* of the illness unfolded (Gerhardt 1989: 160). This was in marked contrast to the temporary nature of illness and treatment in the functionalist perspective, and of 'crisis' in the conflict model. The idea of a 'negotiated order' implied a process of bargaining which could be observed in many different social locales. Indeed, such interactional forms were seen as central to the development of 'modernity' as a whole.

HEALTH, ILLNESS AND SOCIAL CHANGE

Important though the above perspectives have been in medical sociology (and in sociology as a whole) and important though they still are today, much has changed since their formulation in the 1970s. Four aspects of change need to be noted in introducing the topics to be presented in this book. These are: changes in the pattern of illness and the relative growth in the importance of chronic illness; the growing emphasis on *health* in both popular thought and professional practice; changes in the social and economic structures of late modern societies, where professional authority and other key processes concerning self and society are being significantly altered; and changes in medical sociology, where newer perspectives such as feminism and 'postmodernism' have extended and in some cases sought to replace earlier perspectives.

As far as the first of these is concerned, mention has already been made of the growing importance of chronic illness. As will be seen in subsequent chapters, much early medical sociology research was carried out in clinical contexts where acute illness and hospital medical treatment were dominant. Indeed, the clinic was both the focus *and* locus of a number of studies, and provided the context in which the competing sociological perspectives outlined above could be examined. These frequently assumed, however, that acute illness and the clinic were central to the study of health and illness.

However, community-based studies were also beginning to reveal, as was noted above, that much illness did not find its way to the clinic. This view of the 'symptom iceberg' (Hannay 1979) in part gave credence to the study of *illness behaviour* and *help-seeking behaviour*, but it also revealed that much illness had become increasingly chronic in character. Though it could be seen that patients with chronic illness made use of health care at various stages in an unfolding condition, much of its everyday management occurred in the lay setting and without professional assistance.

Underlying this were important changes in the demographic structures of modern societies. When Parsons was writing in the 1950s, acute infectious disease among young adults still dominated much of the lay experience of illness and professional thought in the health care field (although, of course, chronic forms of illness were not unknown). Since then the pattern of illness has changed markedly towards diseases associated with a much older demographic profile in nearly all modern societies – the so-called *demographic transition* (for a discussion of this, see Bury 1988, 1992a). Indeed, the near panic response to the emergence of HIV/AIDS in the 1980s (and then CJD in the 1990s) arose partly from the lack of familiarity with life-threatening infectious diseases in the young, at a time when these had been thought to have almost completely disappeared in Western societies.

Second, in addition to the issues of chronic illness and ageing (and in some tension with them) has been the growing emphasis on *health* in contemporary culture. Though medical care and medical science remain central to modern societies, alongside them has been an increasing emphasis on health and *health promotion*. The cultural shift from a preoccupation with illness to health reflects, in part, as Coward (1989) has pointed out, a developing scepticism towards science and a preference for 'natural' remedies and 'alternative' medical approaches. From this viewpoint 'lifestyle', 'health-related behaviours' and 'health promotion' have all taken on as much importance in recent years as disease prevention and medical intervention did in the first decades following the Second World War.

A 'positive' definition of health has sought to displace a negative medical one, defined as the absence of disease. Questions concerning health-related quality of life and well-being have grown, partly to evaluate the management of chronic illness but also as part of a wide variety of health promotion activities. The increasing salience of these concepts, with related professional activities, signals a relative decline of medical and scientific categories in late modern cultures. Medical sociologists such as Stacey have argued that in such a cultural context, *health* rather than illness and medicine should be the focus of sociological enquiry (Stacey and Homans 1978), though, as will be seen, this is an ambiguous terrain in which to work.

Third, there have been major changes in the nature of social life and the economy more generally, with considerable implications for health and health care. In very broad terms, the 'restructuring' of modern capitalist societies can be seen to involve a marked shift from a preoccupation with production to one of consumption. The service and public sectors now comprise a major part of contemporary economies, displacing industrial production from its central economic role. The development of the 'world economy' has been accompanied within national boundaries by the decline in manufacturing and the rise of consumerist activities (Lash and Urry 1987: 16). In this view, the power of organised labour diminishes and that of 'public opinion' and the 'consumer' rises.

This set of changes is important to the analysis of health, illness and health care. Changes in the economic logic of capitalism mean that the well-established links between social class and illness need to be set against changes in employment patterns and, indeed, the relative decline in the importance of employment as a whole. Structural unemployment, changing gender relations in employment, early retirement and an ageing population all need to be taken into account in assessing evidence on inequalities in health. In turn, health matters throw important light on these economic and social transformations. The future of the welfare state, as well as the analysis of health inequalities (or 'variations', in official circles), is having to be rethought (Baldwin and Falkingham 1994; Burrows and Loader 1994). It is no longer possible to see health systems as 'external' to the capitalist economy.

In health care, restructuring (termed 'reforms' by the British Conservatives in the 1980s) has been proceeding at a rapid pace, particularly with the introduction of the 'internal market' in the National Health Service (Mohan 1991, 1996). This has involved major changes in organisation and outlook in the NHS, in the attempt to move the centre of gravity away from the 'producers' or providers of health care to *patients as consumers*. In the 1970s the idea that patients should be seen as consumers was anathema to medical sociologists such as Stacey (1976) but as the 1980s and 1990s have unfolded the ideology of 'consumerism' has seemed unstoppable. Consumerist ideology also underpins the growth of evaluation and patient-based measures of the outcomes of health care, such as health-related quality of life (Bury 1994a).

This also illustrates a general cultural trend in late modern societies to become more 'reflexive' in character, as people are required to assimilate and evaluate increasing amounts of information, especially about health risks. These processes produce a 'contestable culture' in which trust in abstract systems and expertise is frequently threatened (Giddens 1991). This is particularly true in such matters as health risks from the environment, food production, pharmaceutical products and other medical treatments. All these add to the challenge to dominant modes of thought and practice, including those which have long gone unquestioned in medicine and health care (Gabe *et al.* 1994). The authority of the 'medical model', expressed historically in the emergence of the individualistic doctor–patient relationship in the late nineteenth and early twentieth centuries (Lawrence 1995), is now giving way to more pluralistic forms. A more 'contractual' or 'consumerist' relationship between health care professionals and patients as 'equal partners' may be emerging as a result.

The fourth and final aspect of change which needs to be highlighted is the outlook of medical sociology itself. Much of the impetus for the development of the perspectives of the 1960s and 1970s came from a desire among sociologists to break away from existing 'policy driven' social research, especially that based on 'positivistic' methodologies. Much of the early collaboration between public health academics and medical sociologists was of this nature (Jefferys 1991: 16). Sociologists interested in health were often expected to do little more than add 'social factors' to medical surveys and carry out interviewing.

Today, the intellectual legacy of the 1970s remains of value, but the changes in health and society outlined here have been accompanied, in turn, by the growing influence of different sociological perspectives. The most obvious of these is feminist thought, which, though not new in itself, has in various guises continued to mount effective challenges to the 'gender blind' nature of much traditional sociological research, including that in medical sociology (e.g. Stacey 1988). Though much feminist research in the health field was initially preoccupied with reproductive health, there have recently been calls to extend its scope, for example into the health of older women and men (Arber 1994). Indeed, Arber uses such a perspective to challenge medical sociology to take up the *gendered* character of the ageing population and its associated health dimensions, including those of chronic illness and disability (Arber 1994; Arber and Ginn 1991). Other forms of feminist thought have recently been brought to bear on issues such as the treatment of mental illness (Ettorre and Riska 1995) and measuring outcomes of care (Oakley 1992).

The other main perspective in medical sociology which departs in major respects from the legacy of the past is what is sometimes called 'post-structuralist' or 'postmodernist' theorising (some of it feminist in character), especially that influenced by Foucault. In the depiction of a transition to a 'postmodern society' the unifying categories of culture, social roles, self and identity give way to notions of fragmented and disorganised social relations, of renewed interest in 'multiple realities' and of 'decentred' selves. Much of this sociology has become less concerned with exploring existing theoretical perspectives or gathering reliable and valid data, and more concerned with tracing the links between knowledge and power and the ways language and 'truth claims' constitute reality (including subjectivity).

The shift in cultural emphasis towards consumerism and health rather than illness, together with a more pluralistic medical setting in which self-help groups, media-based information systems and alternative medicine are growing, is helping to constitute the transformation of 'modern' into 'postmodern' society (Hassan 1985). In this perspective the 'modern' expert (white-coated and the source of rational scientific knowledge) is not just being challenged, but is relegated to being merely one of a number of more or less authoritative sources. From this viewpoint, it is argued, medical sociology needs to abandon its intellectual roots and adopt an approach to health and illness which sees them as being constituted through an array of 'discursive practices'. Indeed, even health becomes a 'possibility' rather than a reality (Fox 1993). As result, the values of 'public health' themselves are subject to scrutiny in an attempt to 'undermine and contest accepted understandings and assumptions about public health and health promotional practices' (Lupton 1995: 14).

The issues that are being addressed in these forms of 'postmodernist' sociology are noteworthy, particularly as the balance sheet of modernity is drawn up at the close of the millennium. Various problems are highlighted as a result of such analysis, among them the development of powerful 'surveillance techniques' through medical activity, the nature of health risks including those produced by medicine itself, the need for 'reflexive' assimilation of health information, the importance of gender, age and ethnicity alongside social class, and the impact of a consumer culture on health. These are all matters of concern and are discussed in subsequent chapters of this book. However, the idea that these signify the arrival of a 'postmodern' society requiring a 'postmodern medical sociology', with no value commitment to public health, is more debatable, and constitutes an approach about which there must be reservations.

The view put forward in *Health and Illness in a Changing Society* is that, while there is a need to re-examine the sociological perspectives of the 1970s, care needs to be taken not to overstate the degree of change occurring, or to adopt wholesale forms of 'data free' postmodern speculative thinking. As Giddens has pointed out, the contention that we have entered a 'postmodern' era is to presume that social dislocation and fragmentation (difficult to define, let alone demonstrate) are particularly new or completely dominate experience (Giddens 1991: 27). Such thinking also runs the danger of conveying a cavalier attitude towards the enormous achievements that modern society, including modern (medical) science, has accomplished. For all its problems and deleterious effects, modernity has produced a degree of personal security and material well-being for millions of people, unheard of before in human history. It has also been associated with a form of selfhood based on mutual respect and self-fulfilment; the pursuit of the ideal of 'authenticity' in social relationships (C. Taylor 1991).

Equally important, as Giddens has argued, the 'unifying features' of modern institutions provide new possibilities for life in the future, as well as creating problems. In this sense the term 'high modernity', or perhaps the less flowery 'late modern society', conveys more accurately the tension between the long-term trends of modern life and the transformations now under way. The possibilities and hazards of modernity, nowhere more obvious than in illness, health and medicine, are thus still being worked through. It is impossible accurately to predict the future of these within a sociological frame of reference. A more limited role is to try to make sense of what is happening, as well as to evaluate social trends as they develop. In this process, sociology will need to examine critically, but not throw overboard, the legacy of 'modernist' analysis – and the emphasis on collecting empirical evidence – that it has built up in throughout its history.

There is one last consideration that needs to be borne in mind in thinking about these issues. This is that, for all the changes that are affecting people's lives in modern societies, disease, illness and death still represent a constant reminder of the biological limits of life.

Medical sociology would not be true to its task if it dealt with the suffering and pain that illness involves as if they were mere 'fabrications' of historically or culturally contingent 'discourses'. Changes in thought and practice cannot be critically evaluated without a recognition that one major strand in modern life has been to attempt to reduce suffering and promote the public health. Elusive though this has often been, and while claims to promote well-being through medical intervention have often served the interests of powerful professional groups, it does not detract from the efforts to achieve a better society, which involves good quality health care and medical treatment. The need empirically to evaluate professional interests *and* the achievements of medicine should be at the heart of medical sociology research.

PLAN OF THE BOOK

The topics which comprise the chapters which follow are inevitably a selection from a potentially very wide range. They have been selected on the basis of their continuing importance to medical sociologists and their relevance to modern health care issues. The aim is to provide the reader with a critical review of the relevant literature, combined with an outline of the more recent trends and debates. Selected key words and concepts have been *italicised* in the text (apart from giving emphasis) in order to remind the reader of the *conceptual focus* of sociological research on health and illness. Though some of the literature is covered briefly, some is dealt with at greater length. The variety of *quantitative and qualitative* methods employed in medical sociology research are highlighted where relevant.

Chapter 1 begins by considering the nature of *health beliefs* and *health knowledge* in the development of modern society. Though, as has been noted, much medical sociology research on illness began in the clinic setting, under the influence of anthropological writings the study of *lay beliefs* began to emerge. Health beliefs research has concentrated in two issues: the nature of lay ideas about the *causes* of illness, and beliefs about *personal responsibility* for health. In recent years there has been a stronger emphasis on the nature of *lay knowledge* of both disease and illness, and also of health more generally. These issues are discussed in the context of the rise in health promotion activities and their competition for public adherence with the orthodox medical model of illness. The potential for continuing conflict between lay and professional modes of thought is considered.

In chapter 2, consideration is given to one of the most important debates concerning the social determinants of health, namely that on *inequalities in health*. In this chapter the background to and key arguments of the Black Report, which became the focus of considerable academic and public attention in the early 1980s, are examined. The strengths and weaknesses of the approach adopted in that report are discussed, particularly in the context of important changes in the class structure in Britain and the related emphasis which has now come to the fore on *social position* to include ethnicity and gender. Whilst this debate has been central to showing how health and illness are *socially patterned*, the interpretation of the evidence is less than clear cut. For some, inequalities in health show the urgent need to tackle either poverty or disparities in wealth and income (or both), while for others such differences indicate *acceptable inequalities* or simply *health variations* (to use the term preferred in Conservative health policy) where lay people are seen to exercise choice in health-related behaviours. In this way the political character of the analysis of health inequalities is sharply revealed.

In chapter 3 the book turns to one of the key features of the social responses to and action in illness, namely the *doctor–patient relationship*. This emerged as a central focus of medical sociology research in the 1960s and 1970s, partly as the result of a growing sense of crisis in official circles, especially with respect to relationships and apparent low morale in General Practice in Britain. In recent years, however, the situation has changed considerably. As patients have become less deferential, and as GPs have increasingly worked in teams rather than as isolated individuals, evidence for a more *consumerist* or *contractual* relationship needs to be considered. In addition, as the doctor's role changes, other forms of health care interaction (including those with other professionals such as managers or nurses) potentially take on greater significance.

In chapter 4 the changing patterns of health and illness are illustrated by examining medical sociology's contribution to the study of chronic illness and disability. In this context, the *meaning of illness* alongside studies of the *social patterning of disability* has received particular attention, complementing work on lay health beliefs. The impact of symptoms on daily activities and the wider implications of chronic disorders have been studied in some detail in a range of specific disorders. The *social disruption* associated with such illness has been the focus of much enquiry, as have the efforts lay people make to maintain normal life. These often involve considerable levels of *negotiation* and *self-management* techniques. Recently, this approach has been challenged by disability activists who have criticised both medical and sociological research – the former for medicalising disability and the latter for underestimating the conflictual nature of disability experience in modern societies. The nature of the debate currently being conducted between medical sociologists and disability activists also raises issues concerning the nature of the research process, and is discussed in the latter part of the chapter.

As has been argued, death constitutes the most intense personal and social reality that humans have to face, and this is the focus of chapter 5. Much of the research carried out by medical sociologists in this area has sought to draw attention to what are taken to be the negative consequences of an individualistic medical model. Those writing about death and dying from an historical and sociological viewpoint have pointed to the contradiction of the growth in the hospitalisation of the dying patient at the point when technical medicine, emphasising cure, has been at its height. In such circumstances death appears to be the expression of medical failure, with resulting negative consequences for the dying person and those around them. Research on *awareness contexts* points to the difficulties involved in professional–patient relationships under such circumstances. The advent and growing influence of the hospice movement has signalled considerable change in this area, and the chapter looks at the sociological work that is emerging. In particular, this part of the discussion tries to evaluate the impact of hospice and 'palliative care' on the experience of dying in modern society, and whether it is possible to fashion a *Good Death*.

The final chapter tackles an issue which runs through many of the topics discussed in the book, though not usually explicitly. This concerns *the body*. Research on health beliefs, chronic illness and dying are all implicitly concerned with how human beings deal simultaneously with changes to the body as well as to self and identity. Indeed, it might be argued that *all* discussions of health touch on the subject of the body – the considerations of both *mortality* and individual *death* refer in different ways to the impact of illness on physical survival. In recent years, however, mainstream sociologists and some medical sociologists have been arguing for a more explicit conceptual focus on the body. This, it is held, is necessary in order to provide a more adequate theory of social action as well as understanding a consumer culture which has become preoccupied with *health and risk*. Here, risk may refer to environmental hazard, food contamination, medical treatments or forms of *risk behaviours*.

In this way the discussion of *Health and Illness in a Changing Society* can be concluded, if only provisionally. As has been said, the future is impossible to predict. Whether health will remain a central organising cultural motif of late modern societies in the future, as it has become in the recent past, is difficult to say. And whether new forms of medical science and technology will renew medicine's authority in dealing with illness, or simply add further fuel to an increasingly sceptical public perception, cannot easily be determined. On present evidence health and illness will continue to be tackled at both individual and collective levels in circumstances of considerable uncertainty – as perhaps they have always been. The social and ethical implications of modern medicine will continue to need clear and cogent analysis and evaluation, and making sense of illness in a changing world will continue to be needed as people (whether lay or professional) try to find pathways through the hazardous terrain of late modern life. This is the agenda for future research in medical sociology.

Chapter 1

From illness behaviour to health beliefs and knowledge

INTRODUCTION

This opening chapter traces the emergence of health beliefs as an important part of the medical sociology research agenda. It shows how this has reflected changes in both health policy and the wider culture surrounding health in late modern societies. It is important to recognise at the outset, however, that interest in this area among sociologists of medicine is relatively recent. Gerhardt, for example, in her wide-ranging review of the development of medical sociology discussed in the introduction to this book, deals briefly with 'lay theories' and 'patient views' of illness, but does not give prominence to wider issues of lay beliefs about health and medicine more generally (Gerhardt 1989). As will be seen, until the 1980s sociological interest in behaviour and interaction in the health service setting has tended to overshadow a broader concern with the way lay people view health. It is therefore somewhat ironic that studies of health beliefs by medical sociologists have emerged at a time when the idea of a distinct concept of *lay beliefs* has come in for serious and critical examination, especially by anthropologists. Although the terms 'belief' and 'lay beliefs' are now being used widely in social research on health, they are more problematic than they seem.

A useful starting point in considering these issues and in providing a guide to the chapter is provided by the anthropologist Byron J. Good in his recent book *Medicine, Rationality and Experience* (Good 1994). Good begins by pointing to the long tradition, and ambiguity, in the general anthropological literature on beliefs, especially where these appear to differ from what appears to be self-evidently true to the investigator. In particular, Good argues, problems for anthropologists have arisen when they have been confronted with the gap between beliefs held by peoples in traditional societies and those based on more 'reality congruent' forms of knowledge in modern science-based cultures, from which they, as investigators, have emerged.

Good also argues that, in most of the anthropological canon, the tendency to counterpose lay beliefs against scientific knowledge has meant a failure to provide a clear analysis of their relationship. As a result, anthropology has conveyed the idea that beliefs may be culturally sustained (for example, in the existence of witches) even when they are felt by the investigator to be clearly 'untrue'. Through a detailed discussion of the way in which the term 'belief' and related concepts have developed, Good argues that anthropology has essentially utilised a notion of belief that 'connotes error or falsehood, though it is seldom explicitly asserted' (Good 1994: 17). As a result, the growing importance of the concept of 'belief' has, for Good, been fateful for anthropology.

The answer to this dilemma, for Good, is to focus on the contextual nature of knowledge, whether (in the medical field) that held by scientists and doctors or by 'lay' actors. In this sense, Good echoes the call by Comaroff for all ideas about illness to be treated as features of 'symbolic systems' (Comaroff 1982). Rather than scientific medicine being treated as if it were a 'mirror of nature' it should be regarded, according to these authors, as a 'rich *cultural language* linked to a highly specialised version of reality and system of social relations' including 'deep moral concerns' as well as technical ones (Good 1994: 5, emphasis in original). Similarly, lay practices and interpretations should be studied in order to reveal the 'diverse interpretive practices through which illness realities are constructed, authorized, and contested in personal lives and social institutions' (ibid.).

In so doing, Good is critical of researching beliefs within an 'empiricist' framework, which treats scientific facts as objectively true, and which, he argues, detracts from the central task of explicating the use of language, the fashioning of meanings in relation to experience and the development of 'representations' of ideas about disease and illness in the wider culture. One of the examples he uses in criticising 'empiricist' research is the development by psychologists of a Health Belief Model, through which it is hoped that subjective and cognitive factors can be studied in order to predict behavioural outcomes such as the use of services, and through which 'false beliefs' can be corrected, for the benefit of the public health (Good 1994: 40).

This kind of 'objectivist' approach to health beliefs, for Good, carries the danger that subjective opinions and accounts, which do not predict behaviour or 'have no grounds in disordered physiology and thus objective reality', are taken to be unreal (Good 1994: 10). Beliefs in this context are treated as irrational, and counterposed to rational scientific medical knowledge. Put simply, lay people have beliefs and doctors have knowledge. The basis of a sceptical view of this opposition, Good argues, can derive from the long tradition in anthropology of observing actually occurring cultures in which the absence of Western scientific knowledge is entirely consistent with the existence of viable forms of social life.

The importance of this debate for this opening chapter is that it helps to lay bare a series of tensions to be found in research on health and illness. Opposition between illness and disease, lay beliefs and professional knowledge, subjectivity and objectivity – in short, opposition between the worlds of patients and doctors – has been a major theme in medical sociology. Good argues that each mode of thought and practice should be regarded, relativistically, in its own social context. In this way the form and content of each can receive proper attention. Though this relativism may, in turn, avoid awkward questions of how we evaluate one form of culture against another (Gellner 1992), Good's approach does, at least, point to the real difficulties of maintaining a strict separation between the ideas, beliefs and practices of 'lay people' and the scientifically based knowledge of professional health care workers and 'experts'. In following such a line of argument, however, it is equally important not to fall into the trap of treating all lay ideas as if they are true and expert ideas as inherently suspect. A route out of this dilemma is to pay attention to the social consequences of beliefs (whether lay or professional) within a value framework that has a continuing commitment to the relief of pain and suffering. As will be seen in chapter 6, Good's 'soft relativism' in exploring the lay/professional divide is tempered in this way and by a strong adherence to empirical evidence on the nature of such consequences.

In any event, institutional changes in late modern societies are themselves undermining the maintenance of strict dividing lines and boundaries between lay and professional modes of thought. Not only have critiques of an empiricist science and of depictions of 'irrational' lay ideas emerged to challenge such oppositions, but the social conditions which have sustained these distinctions, and the intellectual positions related to them, have also altered in a number of significant ways.

Again, as argued in the introduction to this book, disease, illness, health and medicine all occur today in a social context of considerable complexity. The development of health promotion, the related but separate processes of the massive information explosion on health and medicine, the decline in the central position of medical authority as the unquestioned source of knowledge and the growth of pluralistic forms of health care, including 'alternative' forms of medicine, all point to the relative decline in the pre-eminence of 'objectivist' science criticised by Good.

The study of health beliefs has therefore turned, in recent years, from a focus on the gulf between lay and scientific modes of thought to one where each is considered in a context of rapid social change. This shifting scene is characterised by considerable overlap and erosion of boundaries. Today, people's *lay knowledge* of health and illness is likely to be studied as much as their *lay beliefs*. However, before developing this argument in more detail, there is first a need to sketch in the influential legacy of the 1970s, in which a clear lay/professional divide was propounded. From there it will be possible to look at the emergence of social research on health beliefs (influenced by the kind of anthropological insights discussed above) and then the further exploration of ideas about lay knowledge.

THE LAY/PROFESSIONAL DIVIDE IN MEDICAL SOCIOLOGY

The origins of the sociological, as opposed to the anthropological, study of health beliefs can be seen in the examination of the issues of *medical dominance, illness behaviour* and *lay referral processes* in the use of medical services. During the 1960s and 1970s a critical analysis of the power of medicine was developed, reacting to the rapid growth in importance of medical thought and practice following the Second World War. This was especially related to the massive increase in medical activity in the US and its expansion in the rest of the 'developed world'. Although, as Strong (1979a) has argued, the critical sociologists were, of course, engaged in seeking greater social influence for themselves in setting out their case, the argument ran that doctors and a ('mechanistic' or 'objectivist') biomedical model were exercising *undue* influence over the organisation of health care and over the lay public in general. Attention to illness behaviour and lay referral processes also aimed to act as a counter-weight to the widespread medical view that patients exhibited irrational tendencies in responding to symptoms, and in deciding whether to use services or not. Doctors routinely complained that patients both delayed seeking help and presented with trivial complaints, especially to GPs' surgeries. These paradoxical injunctions can still be heard emanating from the medical profession today.

The most cogent sociological critique of professional power, at this time, was that of Eliot Freidson (1970a, 1970b). In his influential book, *Profession of Medicine*, Freidson put forward the idea that the world of medicine and doctoring, based on a technical/scientific model of disease, stood in sharp contrast to that of lay persons and patients and their concerns with illness. As a result, Freidson argued, the increasing organisation and extension of modern medicine posed a threat to the civil liberties of modern populations. This was partly because medicine's professional autonomy frustrated proper regulation by the state, and partly because its monopoly over determining what was, and what was not, illness effectively excluded patients' concerns from medical practice. From the dominant medical perspective, patients' perceptions and beliefs were either ignored or rejected out of hand (Freidson 1970a).

In short, Freidson argued, there existed an inherent conflict of perspectives between doctors and patients (Freidson 1970a: 323). In contrast to Parsons' (1951) earlier claim that there was a high degree of reciprocity between doctors and patients, Freidson argued that conflict was built into modern medicine. This, in turn, was based on fundamental differences between the biological and social realms in understanding illness. Freidson stated:

> While illness as a biophysical state exists independently of human knowledge and evaluation, illness as a social state is *created and shaped* by human knowledge and evaluation.
>
> (1970a: 223, emphasis in original)

The main point of this argument was to underline Freidson's contention that illness as a form of social deviance is 'imputed and not merely "there"' (p. 222). Labelling theory, which was developed in the 1960s to provide a critical account of deviance in modern society, could thus be extended to take into account all forms of illness, and not just mental illness, to which it had been applied by writers such as Scheff (1966). This extension, Freidson and his followers hoped, would bring a critical edge to bear on the study of medical practice as a whole. The processes involved in the 'imputation' of illness by doctors, and their institutionalised expression in the modern clinic, where doctors exercised considerable power relative to lay people, led Freidson to argue that:

> while the patient can be involved in mutual participation by virtue of his [sic] similarity to the therapist, he is never wholly co-operative. Given the viewpoints of the two worlds, lay and professional, in interaction, they can never be wholly synonymous. And they are always, if only latently, in conflict.
>
> (Freidson 1970a: 321)

While the main focus of Freidson's work was more concerned with the analysis of medical work and developing a critique of professional autonomy than it was with lay conceptions of illness, this approach opened the way to a greater recognition of the place of the patient and of lay views. An important space opened up in which a more relativistic analysis could be developed in which patients' views could be examined in their own right. Note here, however, that at this time when the lay/professional divide was discussed it was mostly patients' views of *illness* rather than their beliefs about *health* that were under consideration. Problems associated with the treatment of illness rather than the promotion of health dominated the policy and research agendas, and most sociologists at this time were concerned with observing doctors and patients in the context of the hospital or clinic, rather than the broader canvas of everyday life in the community. As argued above, the shift towards a more explicit concern with health beliefs in medical sociology coincided with a growing crisis in modern medical practice and health care systems, and a change towards health promotion policies.

Observational studies dominated the emerging medical sociology research agendas in the UK in the 1970s and were concerned with examining medical dominance and 'lay experiences' of *patients* within the medical encounter. Bloor (1976), for example, studied the 'decision rules' involved in the imputation of the diagnosis of tonsillectomy in patients in ENT clinics, and showed the way in which lay views were effectively ignored or circumvented by the routines employed by doctors. Similarly, Strong studied the 'ceremonial order of the clinic' and the 'bureaucratic format' through which decisions in hospital paediatric services exercised 'powerful control over the shape and content of medical consultations' (Strong 1979b: 212). Though following Freidson's views on the power of the medical profession and the lay/professional divide, Strong attempted to finesse this approach by stressing the complexities of medical encounters, and the use of ceremony and 'medical gentility', as part of maintaining control over the patient. Strong's work was influenced as much by Goffman's 'micro sociology' of interactional rules as by Freidson's rendition of labelling theory. The hospital had become a convenient focus for sociologists' concern with examining the ways in which 'negotiated order' could be constructed in modern societies (Strauss et al. 1963).

The other related concern in sociological research during this period was with debates about access to and utilisation of health care. Here, sociologists also sought to challenge the dominant medical perception of the 'proper' or 'appropriate' use of services by asking what led people to seek help in the first place. The medical approach seemed to rest on the assumption that people should be educated just enough to recognise symptoms correctly and actively seek help at the right time, and then become passive again once in the doctor's surgery, ready to comply with 'doctors' orders' (Bloor and Horobin 1975; Stimson 1974). By contrast, sociologists were keen to situate such help-seeking action in the contexts and social circumstances of people's lives. Again, it was hoped that such work would show that lay people's actual perceptions and actions contained a greater degree of rationality than doctors were prepared to admit, and that ideas of 'educating' patients about appropriate conduct, and bringing them in line with professional dictates, were largely misplaced.

David Mechanic's earlier work had identified a series of factors that might explain lay people's *illness behaviour*. These included lay perceptions concerning the seriousness of symptoms, competing needs such as work or home life and the availability and perceived benefits of services (Mechanic 1968, 1978). This approach was grist to the theoretical mill of writers such as Freidson, in that it showed that patients' concerns were likely to be quite different to those of practitioners who only see illness 'within the purview of the professional sector' (Freidson 1970a: 270). From a sociological perspective, lay concerns about consultation were seen to be influenced by both cultural factors and the nature of local social networks, what

Freidson referred to as the *lay referral system*. Where a social group's cultural outlook was 'incongruent' with that of doctors, and where their social network was 'cohesive' (or 'tight-knit'), a low level of service use (or *utilisation*) was predicted. People in such circumstances tended to rely on their own resources rather than professional help. Conversely, where people shared the dominant medical view of illness and had loose-knit social networks, relying more on friends than family, utilisation was predicted to be high.

Subsequent empirical research – for example, McKinlay's work on the use of ante-natal services in Scotland (McKinlay 1973) – attempted to show that social networks did, indeed, influence service use, along the lines suggested by Freidson. However, although the presence of tight-knit networks appeared to explain low utilisation, the different levels of service use in McKinlay's data were also associated with whether or not the woman was having a first or subsequent child. Low utilisation was particularly associated with women having a second or third child, suggesting that lay referral processes and perceptions of services might be less important than an increase in personal knowledge and self-confidence, gained through experience over time. Moreover, later research by Scambler *et al.* (1981), on women's use of primary care services, showed, in contrast to McKinlay, that those who consulted family members more than friends used services more frequently. Research on lay perceptions and the role of lay networks did not, therefore, shown any consistent influence in service use. Despite this, these studies revealed the importance of the everyday worlds of lay people and the variations in their views and experiences of health-related matters. They also began to shift attention away from a preoccupation with the supposed problems created by a dominant medical model and medical profession within the health care sector, by paying more direct attention to those factors that influenced lay thought and action.

The main point of much of this work was to stress the rational nature of lay help-seeking behaviour, when it was set within specific local contexts. A further example of research from this period illustrates this 'contextual' approach. In a small-scale study in South Wales, Robinson (1971, 1973) asked families to keep health diaries for a month, recording any symptoms experienced and any action taken. The results showed that people had tried and tested ways of dealing with illness and judging when to seek professional help. Robinson's argument was that people did not respond to each illness episode by thinking through and weighing up all the evidence on alternative courses of action. Mothers 'put antiseptic cream on grazed knees, took aspirin for a headache, kept children in the house when they had chills, or called in the doctor when someone's temperature was found to be 102. These mothers knew what to do and did it' (Robinson 1973: 42). Although there was often variation in responses to symptoms between families, this did not mean that people behaved in non-rational ways. Robinson commented that: 'someone may hold a belief without continually assessing evidence and drawing conclusions' (ibid.). Help-seeking behaviour was therefore portrayed as a matter of managing two sets of demands which balanced beliefs and actions in specific circumstances: the demands of everyday life and the demands of the medical services.

At the same time as this work was being conducted in Britain, Irving Zola, in a series of papers based on field studies with different groups of patients in New York, underlined both the variability in the use of services and the cultural dimensions of symptom perception together with the decision to seek help. Contextual factors were also identified that might push people towards or keep people away from services. In an influential paper Zola (1973) identified several triggers that might affect whether people would seek help or not. These included interpersonal crises, disruptions to occupational roles, the importance of 'sanctioning' where a person is allowed or pressurised to consult by others, and 'temporalising', where a time limit is put on tolerating symptoms, to help in deciding whether to consult. Such contextual factors put variations in help-seeking behaviour again in a rational light, setting them within the actual circumstances and constraints of everyday life.

While studies of help-seeking behaviour and decision-making began to focus attention on lay beliefs and actions, in many ways they remained close in outlook to observational studies of lay/professional encounters in clinics. Both were essentially concerned with the processes of 'becoming a patient', either in decision-making on whether to consult or not or in what actually happened in the health service setting. The adoption of an interactionist perspective in order to help understand such processes reflected the desire among medical sociologists to move beyond the 'medical dominance' approach of Freidson as well as the functionalism of Parsons. As elsewhere in sociology, researchers were looking for new approaches to social life, especially those which stressed the different facets of how people could be seen as 'active agents'. In Britain, for example, Dingwall developed an argument about becoming ill which drew on both 'ethnomethodology' and formalistic approaches of linguistic anthropology in tackling the question of agency (Dingwall 1976).

However, despite these developing trends in thinking about illness, there was little sociological research being conducted at this point among healthy populations outside of the help-seeking context. While new theoretical perspectives were being adopted in analysing illness there was little inquisitiveness about the nature of health. Medical sociologists were preoccupied with theoretical and methodological debates but often appeared to be unaware of the policy context in which research was taking place. As argued earlier, research reflected, in most part, the health care agenda of the period, which was concerned with the role of hospital treatment of illness. Policy was especially concerned with the growing size, costs and influence of the acute sector, its proper use and the unintended consequences that its rapid expansion might be creating. Research on primary care and the development of health centres (Jefferys and Sachs 1983) was part of an attempt to move health care away from the over-emphasis on hospitals. There was a fear of an over-reliance on specialised medical treatment, leading to the 'medicalisation of life' in which patienthood would almost become the norm (Zola 1972). This fear was fed by a picture of an increasingly 'high tech' and economically demanding hospital-based medical profession (Illich 1975).

Of interest in this connection is the fact that although medical sociologists in this period were keen to bring the lay/professional divide into the critical light of day, much of the financial support for the research came from official funding bodies including, in Britain, the Department of Health. Governments were keen to know what was happening in the expanding Health Service, particularly whether patients were likely to create a level of demand which would outstrip supply. Popular critiques of modern medicine, such as those by Illich, were taken seriously in official circles. Research on illness behaviour and the encounters between doctors and patients in clinics provided a window on such developments. In many respects the results of such research were largely reassuring for the authorities, though they may not have liked the critical edge and sociological language that the research produced. The point was, however, that people were shown as relying on lay networks for help, and did not appear to be particularly demanding with respect to the services themselves. Sociological research thus helped to create a watchful and reassuring eye over the rapidly expanding medical services. Larger-scale surveys showed that only a small proportion of people sought help in the face of symptoms (Wadsworth *et al.* 1971), and that patients were modest in their demands and deferential in their demeanour towards doctors (Cartwright 1967). Research on the lay/professional divide was therefore not only becoming well established but of increasing interest to policy makers.

Sociology was also given opportunities to research these issues through encouragement from those working in academic public health circles (at that time called 'community medicine' in Britain), who had a wider concern with disease and illness and were keen, in any case, to expand their own critique of dominant patterns of medical practice, which had led to their exclusion from the centre of medical power (Jefferys 1991). The interest of sociologists, there-fore, in applying theoretical insights on social behaviour and interaction in the health service field, coincided with official and professional concerns with the effects of a period of rapid health service development. This helps to explain the relatively large-scale development of medical sociology in Britain compared with other European countries during the period.

However, as this research developed, a more explicit concern with lay beliefs in everyday community settings began to emerge. A shift in concerns from illness to health could be discerned as both researchers and policy makers developed a more questioning approach to the role of the acute medical sector. Public scepticism towards the expanding medical arena was also slowly developing, alongside existing attachments to the acute medical services. Research began to connect with the development of illness preven-tion and health education policies (given a particular boost in 1976 by the then Labour government's support for a more preventive approach, DHSS 1976) and the development of subjective health assessments. However, before discussing these connections in more detail, it is important first to identify some of the main examples of sociological research on lay beliefs about health which marked this transition.

THE EMERGENCE OF HEALTH BELIEFS IN MEDICAL SOCIOLOGY

Perhaps one of the most influential pieces of work on health beliefs to emerge in the early 1970s was that conducted in France by Claudine Herzlich (1973). Though she was keen to link her research to the theme of medical dominance, and thus Freidson's Weberian view of the medical profession's control over work practices and knowledge, this was not her main concern. Herzlich was keen to draw on anthropological insights and a Durkheimian sociology which suggested that the *social representations* of illness and health could be studied in their own right, particularly as they were drawn upon by individuals in specific social contexts. A Durkheimian perspective on such matters underlined the way in which 'collective representations' contributed to the maintenance of social order: that is, 'the mechanism by which the representation becomes established and its function in orientating behaviour' (Herzlich 1973: 12). Hence, if illness was an institutionalised role then individuals' 'conceptions of the situation' must relate to it in systematic ways (Herzlich 1973: 10).

The cultural repertoires of health comprising such conceptions were, in an industrial society, bound to be influenced by medical categories and the doctor–patient relationship, but, Herzlich argued, they also provided a window on specifically lay ideas about the causation of illness and on moral dimensions of people's beliefs. For example, the ways in which illness meant 'bad' and 'health' meant good could be shown (Herzlich 1973: 12). Here, the focus was not so much on people becoming patients, but on lay ideas among the population more generally. Specifically, attention was paid to lay beliefs about the *causes* of disease and illness and what the elusive idea of *health* itself meant.

Herzlich's study involved interviews with 80 middle-class respondents; 68 mostly professional people in Paris and 12 middle-class individuals from a Normandy village. In answering the main question put to them about where they thought illness and disease came from, Herzlich's respondents emphasised both the 'way of life' and the characteristics of individuals. The 'way of life', especially in the city, was seen to 'generate' illness in the form of germs or accidents, but also more generally to make people more prone to mental illness and diseases such as cancer. Preventive action or cure were seen as important, but the 'way of life' that affected individuals in modern society was seen to be largely working against health (Herzlich 1973: 23).

The attributes of individuals, on the other hand, could more readily produce or maintain health, through, for example, a person's nature or temperament. Predisposition and heredity might also play a part in maintaining health or contributing to illness, but the sources of disease and illness were firmly located in the social environment. Herzlich summarised this part of her argument as follows:

> The unhealthy, unnatural constraining society brings man illness. This is a common theme of our analyses, the thread which binds them together.
>
> (Herzlich 1973: 38)

Herzlich then went on to identify the main conceptions of positive health found in the accounts of in her sample. Echoing Freidson's views of medical dominance concerning the 'imputation' of illness, this part of her argument is developed by stating that 'the concept of health, in principle, is of little concern to the doctor; from a practical point of view only illness counts' (Herzlich 1973: 55). However, in contrast with Freidson, Herzlich did not regard lay people's views as being eclipsed by an all-powerful medical profession.

When looked at in depth, Herzlich argued, lay views of health emerge as quite distinct. Three main forms or representations of health are identified in the study, *health-in-a-vacuum, reserve of health* and *health as equilibrium* – see Table 1.1. The last is perhaps the most familiar, with its idea of balance (see Nordenfelt 1993 for a more recent view of health as equilibrium). Health-in-a-vacuum denotes an absence of illness, and indeed a lack of self-consciousness or awareness of the body. The 'reserve of health', on the other hand, draws on notions of constitution and temperament, but also suggests ways in which it can be improved. Herzlich states that: 'This capital asset of vitality and strength may increase or dissipate in the course of time, like all capital' (Herzlich 1973: 57).

Though people were able to provide clear ideas about health in the study, this did not mean that the concepts were always clearly distinguishable from illness. As Table 1.1 also shows, lay concepts of health contain factual, relational, normative and even moral components.

Herzlich argues that in this matrix two main points can be seen. First, people have a clear view of the organic (we might now say

Table 1.1 Lay views of health

	Health-in-a-vacuum	Reserve of health	Equilibrium
	Being	Having	Doing
Content	Absence of positive content	Robustness and strength Resistance to attacks	Physical well-being Good humour Activity Good relations with others
Relation to person	Impersonal fact All or nothing	Personal characteristic Measurable, variable and permanent Secondary awareness	Personal norm All or nothing Immediate awareness
Relation to other forms	—	Basis of equilibrium	Based on reserve of health
Relation to illness	Destroyed by illness	Resistance to illness	Assimilation of disorders

Source: Herzlich 1973: 63

'embodied' or 'corporeal') dimension in a view of health as absence of illness, as shown in the left-hand column. On the other hand, 'health is defined as a mode of relation of the individual to the environment' with an emphasis on physical and social integrity, as shown in the centre and right-hand columns.

Subsequent sociological work on health beliefs, much of it influenced by Herzlich's ideas, has tended to confirm her general line of argument that health resides, for many lay people, within the individual (as a form of 'reserve stock') and that sources of illness lie outside. It is equally clear that the coherence of lay health beliefs, even within specific segments of the cultural order of modern societies, has to be set against their loosely organised and fluid character. Attempts in some academic circles, most notably, as discussed earlier, among psychologists, to establish a Health Belief

Model which will predict health behaviour, have come in for sustained criticism in recent years from this point of view (e.g. Radley 1994: 53–55). As with work on illness behaviour and lay referral processes undertaken by sociologists, the complexities of social and personal factors and the wide range of phenomena grouped together under the umbrella of 'health and illness' militate against any simple explanatory framework. Herzlich's matrix attempted to take this into account by combining the form and content of lay people's beliefs.

What seems to be clear, however, is that in reflecting on health and facing actual episodes of illness people have available cultural repertoires (one might visualise them in the form of 'pull down menus') in order to frame accounts and responses to events. Health beliefs are not invented anew by individuals on each occasion in which they arise, nor are they a set of rigid 'predispositions'. They are relatively stable entities, though reformulated and altered as events unfold over time or as new information is fed in. As Herzlich showed, people's views of health articulate the relationship between the individual and his or her social group within a specific biographical and social context. Other studies have confirmed this view of stable, if complex, health beliefs, and the ability of people clearly to articulate them.

Research in British medical sociology along these lines began to appear in the early 1980s. Blaxter, for example, studied women's beliefs about the causation of disease, but this time among working-class respondents in a Scottish community (Blaxter 1983). As part of a wider project (Blaxter and Paterson 1982) the study found that disease was seen to be caused by a variety of external agents, including germs and viruses, but was also influenced by such factors as 'familial weaknesses' and stresses that might leave a person prone to illness. Thus disease was a phenomenon that a person 'has, gets or catches', in these women's accounts. Blaxter states that the women found it difficult 'to believe that disease was either random or their own responsibility' (Blaxter 1983: 69). Although the causal agents for illness were often 'outside the clinical system' (ibid.) the women's beliefs tied together their past experience and identity in terms of their current bodily experiences. Though the content of health beliefs might be at variance with *current* medical thinking, Blaxter argued that problems can arise if 'the considerable sophistication in the concepts of even poorly educated patients is under-rated' (ibid.).

Blaxter's subsequent large-scale national survey of health and lifestyle underlined the importance of age as well as social class influences on lay beliefs about health in general and not just on ideas about disease causation (Blaxter 1990). In this survey older people stressed a *functional capacity* view of health, in which the ability to carry out everyday tasks was seen as the basis of good health. As with Williams' study of older Aberdonians (R. Williams 1990) Blaxter's study also underlined the moral dimensions of lay views about health, as suggested by Herzlich. Younger people stressed vitalistic and athletic views of health, in which keeping fit was related to a greater sense of personal responsibility for health (Blaxter 1990: 30), whereas older people stressed the ability to remain independent. Gender also differentiated views in this study, with younger men emphasising the more 'athletic' component, and younger women the 'vitalistic' one (ibid.). However, as in her earlier study, the harshness of social conditions was seen by Blaxter to cut across positive conceptions of health. In this way the 'social patterning' of health beliefs, and not just their general form, was explored more fully.

Having said this, it is important not to overplay the existence of a separate set of consistent lay 'health beliefs' (or a range of beliefs) in sharp contrast with medical knowledge – to repeat Good's point, as if lay people have 'beliefs' while doctors have 'knowledge'. In Blaxter's earlier paper (Blaxter 1983) it was also shown that views of the causation of ill health were not markedly different in terms of their logic from those held in medicine, though discrepancies in content could be found. Although people were able to articulate definite beliefs about the sources of health and illness, somewhat paradoxically they often underplayed the role of environment and social factors compared with Herzlich's middle-class respondents. This suggests that 'environmentalist' or social explanations have a stronger currency among those groups closer, culturally, to official, scientific and academic sources of information.

In recent papers (1992, 1993) Blaxter has gone on to discuss the challenge these findings pose for medical sociology. For, despite an emphasis on resisting personal responsibility for health among some of her Scottish respondents, Blaxter has also emphasised that individualistic explanations (in which self-blame for illness occurs) are to be found among many sections of modern communities, including poorer ones. The 'Thatcherite' culture of the 1980s, with its emphasis on individualism, can be seen to have reinforced this aspect of people's thinking. Blaxter argues that respondents in her qualitative study had a firm adherence to the 'Protestant ethic' and a wish to present a moral identity (Blaxter 1993: 138–139).

The reluctance to entirely blame the environment can also be explained by the understandable tendency of people to resist identifying themselves as the victims of circumstance. This may be much easier for sociologists to articulate than people who actually live in difficult conditions. But it is also partly because, when viewed within a temporal or biographical framework, people have a strong tendency to emphasise change and improvement over time, and thus to contrast favourably their health today with that of previous generations (Blaxter 1993: 128). This kind of lay 'optimistic bias' about health may help lay people to retain positive views of both self and others under difficult social conditions. In this sense, sociological work on inequalities in health which constantly stresses the poor health of working-class groups in particular (see chapter 2) clashes with lay ideas and everyday experience of health as a positive attribute, or at least as the capacity to 'carry on' or 'cope' in functional terms.

The move away, as it were, from a 'Freidsonian' view of illness to a 'Herzlichian' view of health has, therefore, uncovered a new set of tensions for medical sociology. As has been shown, the study of patients' views and actions in relation to medical services and settings sought to reveal the play of medical power. This argument was relatively easy to make. After all, few – even physicians – would deny that the medical profession has exerted considerable influence on health care in modern times. Those from very different political persuasions and different social positions, including policy makers, were able to recognise the force of the arguments about the lay/professional divide. To this extent, critiques of medical dominance played to the gallery, as critics such as Strong had implied (Strong 1979a). Moreover, the hierarchical nature of the hospital or clinic was evident enough, to doctor, patient and researcher alike. Not surprisingly, sociological observers were able to find plenty of evidence of the differences in power between the lay and professional worlds.

The study of lay beliefs in the community, however, now exposed medical sociology to more awkward findings. It appeared that lay people (and especially working-class people) had far more individualistic and less social or political views about health than might have been expected in the light of arguments about the 'clash of perspectives' between lay and professional outlooks. The challenge that this posed was that lay concepts of health were far less clear cut than the legacy of unwarranted 'medical dominance' predicted.

This more complex picture became evident at a time when governments in countries such as the UK were increasingly emphasising individual responsibility in health policies, partly in an attempt to limit medical expansion and expenditure. Mention has already been made of the important cultural and political emphasis on individualism by successive Conservative governments, which provided the context and spur for such policy development. By the late 1980s promoting health rather than treating illness was now the official watchword, echoing long-standing criticisms by public health academics and sociologists that the Health Service was, in reality, an 'illness service'. As a result, disease prevention and health education (later broadened to be encompassed by 'health promotion' strategies and a renewed emphasis on primary care) received greater policy attention. Though sociologists had argued that research should be redirected away from medicine to health (Stacey and Homans 1978) the development of individualistic health education strategies in official circles suggested that this terrain might turn out to be more ambiguous than anticipated. Earlier medical concerns about the 'irrational' use or over-use of services could fairly easily be challenged by observing and reporting what patients said and did in the face of symptoms. In a culture now dominated by a massive expansion of health-related information and messages, new and more complex ideological and cultural contexts were emerging within which the study of health beliefs and lifestyles, among the healthy as well as the ill, needed to be interpreted. Preoccupations with demystifying the importance of medical power and medical dominance in clinics and hospitals were being superseded by a complex set of relationships between health beliefs, lifestyle and a fast-changing society.

HEALTH BELIEFS AND HEALTH PROMOTION

One of the main effects of this developing cultural and policy context for research on health beliefs has been the growing need to study the up-take of health promotion and preventative services such as screening. Herzlich was concerned with the fundamental 'representations' of health and health beliefs in a modern culture and a research strategy which built up a picture of these from an inductive exploration of lay ideas. Recent work in Britain, however, has developed in a much more 'policy relevant' if not 'policy driven' context (Gabe *et al.* 1991). Thus, studies of illness behaviour, of the sort promoted by the work of Mechanic, have now been supplemented with a demand for studies of *health behaviour*. As a result, a new tension exists as research is required to help health promoters target services and effect behavioural change. Such research now has to balance attempts to reduce exposure to risk factors such as smoking and 'unsafe' sex with trying to avoid reinforcing the dominant (and as we have seen, individualistic) ideological bias in official thinking about health.

It is perhaps worth repeating at this point that the emphasis on individual responsibility for health and the need to adopt healthy lifestyles was given a particular fillip in the late 1970s by the Labour government's report *Prevention and Health: Everybody's Business* (DHSS 1976). This much-cited report set the scene for subsequent official enthusiasm for healthy lifestyles, especially during the years of Conservative governments following Labour's defeat in 1979. Throughout the 1980s successive ministers of health in the UK, most notably Edwina Currie, made much of the supposed benefit to the nation's health, and the government's exchequer, of following the golden rules of no smoking, sensible or no alcohol consumption, a healthy diet and plenty of exercise. Medical care was not the only, or even the main, source of protecting health, and doctors' autonomy in developing new treatments could not be sustained at any price. Populist political sentiments, challenging professional privileges, were thus combining with a growing culture of 'healthism' (Crawford 1980). Here, however, the charge that the Health Service was an 'illness service' came from the radical right rather than the left, and signalled a marked change in the political climate surrounding research.

The work of Roisin Pill and colleagues is instructive in this context, since it attempted to grapple with these issues as the policy and cultural context changed. In early exploratory work in South Wales, Pill and Stott (1982) examined the lay beliefs and sense of personal responsibility for health among a small sample of 41 working-class women. Like Blaxter, Pill and Stott found that there was a strong preference (at least in the views proffered to the interviewers) for seeing health in terms of 'extrinsic' factors such as 'germs', though the vulnerability of some individuals to specific illnesses was also noted. However, a moral dimension to lay beliefs was evident, in that women in the study did see people as culpable if they failed to look after themselves or took unnecessary risks. Fatalistic attitudes were also frequently expressed as well. In sum:

about half the sample did not refer to the individual's day to day lifestyle choices in their discussion about illness causation.

(Pill and Stott 1982: 48)

The general findings of the survey seemed to suggest that there was a significant gap between lay beliefs and the growing official ideology, with respect to personal responsibility for health.

At the same time, Pill and Stott noted some key differences amongst their sample. It appeared that poorer respondents living in rented accommodation, at that time mainly local authority housing, were more likely to express fatalistic attitudes or to be resistant to ideas of individual responsibility than respondents who were in more secure employment and buying their own homes, even though they were all nominally from the same social class background. The home owners were more likely to identify with official messages about health, as part of a 'socially mobile' lifestyle. A further paper (Pill and Stott 1985) developed this analysis and argument further, but cast some doubt on the picture of poorer people having fatalistic beliefs and better-off people having more optimistic ones. It appeared that a sense of individual responsibility was more widespread than had initially been observed.

One of the questions which arose from this work concerned the relationship between beliefs as stated in the interviews and actual behaviour. The relationship between belief and behaviour is, of course, rarely a straightforward matter. In a more recent paper (Pill, Peters and Robling 1993) the links between health beliefs and risk behaviour were explored in more depth, by comparing data from their own South Wales studies and a subset of working-class women respondents from Blaxter's (1990) national *Health and Lifestyles* survey, which has already been discussed. Pill *et al.* focused on health behaviours, following the work carried out in the US in the Almeda County Study (Berkman and Breslow 1983). This involved the use of a research instrument comprising 1 or 0 scores for the following: never having smoked; no/moderate use of alcohol; regular exercise; eating breakfast regularly; not snacking between meals; regularly sleeping 7–8 hours each night; and being the correct weight for one's height. The scores from each of these dimensions were then summed into the *Health Practice Index* (HPI) (Pill *et al.* 1993: 1138).

In comparing the data sets, two main findings with respect to the HPI emerged. The first was that in the Cardiff data, but not in the national *Health and Lifestyles* study, education level was significantly associated with higher HPI scores. That is, when further or higher education was present among the working-class women in Cardiff, this was associated with the adoption of a set of 'healthy behaviours', though this was not replicated in the national study. However, when housing tenure was examined in both studies it was found to be highly significant, as in their previous research. The authors stated that:

> Mothers in rented accommodation . . . are significantly less likely than those buying their own houses to report low risk health behaviours.
>
> (Pill *et al.* 1993: 1143)

The authors go on to conclude that the causal direction of associations between the variables in these findings cannot be assumed. Interpreting the links between factors such as home ownership and health behaviours requires, they suggest, further research based on more fine-grained qualitative research techniques. The use of social survey data of the sort they present 'follows the traditional epidemiological model of research' (ibid.). Frequently this means that questions about the meaning of events being reported are dealt with after the data are collected, rather than as part of the study design.

While this suggests the continuing need for carefully conducted sociological research on the relationship between beliefs and behaviour, the earlier part of the paper deals with issues that arise as the result of the policy context of the research. Here, ideology rather than methodology is at stake, and it is these difficulties that are particularly relevant to the current discussion. The authors argue that the rationale for the kind of research they are reporting on is that:

> In order to design more effective programmes it is necessary to be able to identify target groups or individuals who need special attention [and to provide] guidance about potential 'levers' that could be the focus of intervention studies.
>
> (Pill *et al.* 1993: 1137)

It may be persuasively argued that applied medical sociology research should make a positive contribution to shaping such policy goals, but there is clearly a danger here that research on health beliefs and behaviour may become caught up in the pursuit of government policy, and even in attempts to directly engineer the behaviour of groups deemed to be at risk. Though changing people's health behaviours may well be thought to be justified from a public health view, especially with regard to the poorer health record of 'lower-class groups', a critical view of health promotion strategies is also important. Without this the constraints that social contexts and circumstances exert over individuals' behaviour may be lost from view. Moreover, such an approach may help in 'blaming the victim' (Crawford 1977) or act as a source of 'ideological succour' to the socially mobile. Indeed these were matters which were recognised as problematic in Pill and Stott's earlier papers.

Much depends, in this area as in others, on what questions are selected and what are left out of the research. The above research concentrated on selected behaviours, many of which have a strongly normative flavour, such as 'not snacking between meals', or maintaining 'correct weight', around which social values may vary. In this sense, the research questions already embodied social values, which arguably might have been examined as part of the research process rather than presumed by it.

In contrast, in a small-scale exploratory study reported by Calnan and Johnson (1985) and Calnan (1987), an attempt was made to include a wider range of ideas about responsibility for health alongside those of the individual, offsetting the tendency to focus entirely on individual 'risk behaviours'. Whilst respondents in this study were asked about their own role in maintaining health, the responsibilities of doctors (here, general practitioners) and the government in protecting health were also examined.

At first sight, respondents in this study seemed to give expression once more to the dominant idea of individual responsibility for health. Calnan states that 'all the women showed that the responsibility primarily lay with the individual' (Calnan 1987: 87). However, Calnan goes on to argue that this appeared to be a 'surface view', suggesting that *social acceptability* may govern responses to questions about public matters, and may vary from private sentiments (Cornwell 1984). It is worth noting here that the tendency for people to under-report 'undesirable behaviour' has long been seen as a problem in sociological research (Lee 1993: 99). By changing the line of questioning other responses may be elicited. When the women in Calnan's study were asked, for example, what part the government had to play in helping to keep people healthy, a range of views emerged, including an emphasis on regulating drinking and driving. Here too, however, middle-class respondents emphasised personal liberty and the need to limit government action on health education (Calnan 1987: 89).

The implications of this argument are important, if only in reinforcing the point that research on health beliefs can easily slip into reflecting and reinforcing dominant views that need more careful evaluation. Exploring the range of 'cultural repertoires' that people may draw upon in responding to official health messages and the constraints over the adoption of 'healthy behaviours' (on smoking, see, for example, Graham 1993) provides researchers with the potential to examine the social patterning of beliefs and lifestyle *and* their ideological dimensions (Calnan 1994). A more critical as well as an applied perspective can thus be constructed. The final section of this chapter considers an example of recent research on health beliefs exemplifying such an approach, and comes from the work of Davison and colleagues, again working in South Wales.*

HEALTH BELIEFS AND LAY EPIDEMIOLOGY

Davison *et al.*'s discussion of health beliefs focuses on a specific area of health promotion and disease prevention, namely coronary heart disease (Davison *et al.* 1991, 1992). Research on everyday perceptions of heart disease was carried out in a setting where a vigorous health promotion campaign – Heartbeat Wales – had been running during the period of fieldwork. This campaign embodied much of the official thinking on health promotion discussed above, with an emphasis on individual healthy lifestyles, though the campaign did undertake work with local organisations, for example with local food stores in promoting 'healthy eating'. Davison's study was based on extensive interviewing and observations with people in 'naturalistic settings'; in homes, work places and in public areas. The basic aim of the study was to uncover the structure and content of lay health beliefs – especially about lifestyle – in a context of considerable local and national information production and dissemination, and to compare these with the assumptions built into

* This section draws upon a wider discussion of health promotion ideology in Bury (1994b).

official thinking on health promotion, embodied in campaigns such as Heartbeat Wales.

The results of Davison's interviews and observations showed that popular beliefs included an emphasis on individual responsibility for health. People in the study expressed agreement with some of the main lines of the 'healthy behaviour' approach, especially in areas such as smoking and control of weight. Indeed, being obese was identified by respondents in this study as one of the main characteristics of becoming a potential 'candidate' to suffer from heart disease. From this viewpoint, and as with Pill and Stott and Blaxter's work, there is widespread acceptance of the idea that a large measure of choice can be exercised in being and remaining healthy, and that people to some extent bring illness on themselves (Davison *et al.* 1991: 23).

Lay ideas and beliefs about health and illness within contemporary settings can often, therefore, be seen to overlap with those emanating from professional sources. Indeed, in the current cultural context it is sometimes difficult to tell where ideas or knowledge originate. In the case of Heartbeat Wales, the slogan 'The healthy choices are the easy choices' both expressed and reinforced already existing lay beliefs about heart disease. In such a climate, Freidson's idea of a major 'clash of perspectives', between the lay and professional spheres, has limited application. However, Davison makes it clear that individuals continue to draw on ideas about health that do diverge and conflict, to some extent, with official thinking.

It is here that the notion of 'lay epidemiology' comes into play. What Davison has in mind, in coining this term, relates to the 'pull down memory' metaphor used earlier in this chapter. For most of the time 'health' is usually a taken-for-granted feature of everyday life, and may not be a significant issue (Calnan 1994: 74). But when ill health occurs people have to step back from everyday realities and reflect on its effects on others, or on themselves. Under such circumstances Davison *et al.* argue that individuals respond in part by drawing on the 'knowledge and lore received from the wider society' (Davison *et al.* 1991: 5). As noted with respect to Blaxter's work, such information is transmitted horizontally, across social groups, and over time, between generations and throughout the life course. *Lay knowledge* of health and illness, as it is experienced in communities, is then used to fashion encounters with misfortune and illness in the present.

The boundary between 'lay beliefs' and 'lay knowledge' becomes difficult to disentangle, as people observe the occurrence of illness and derive from these observations relatively stable views of those factors which influence it. Just as official epidemiology is concerned with the occurrence and distribution of disease and illness in populations, so lay thinking is concerned with making sense of illness episodes, usually within the more immediate settings of family and community (for broader aspects of the politics of 'lay epidemiology' and the environment see G. Williams and Popay 1994, and P. Brown 1995). New information, for example from health promotion campaigns, is then evaluated against this 'lay epidemiology'. Alongside the elements of individual behaviour and choice, the South Wales study found, importantly, that people have developed ideas about the *social circumstances* surrounding the occurrence of illness, and draw on more *fatalistic ideas* when either personalistic or social types of explanation seem inadequate. It is worth filling out some of the detail here.

In terms of the social components of health, respondents in the South Wales study identified a wide range of circumstances and environmental factors that might promote ill health. In addition to individual behaviour, factors such as stress and strain at work, financial worries and poor working conditions were all reported to play a part in the occurrence of coronary heart disease. Such was the range of factors alluded to by people in the study that Davison comments, 'One of the striking aspects of this width is that almost any type of person could be a candidate (for heart disease)' (Davison *et al.* 1991: 13).

As can be seen in Table 1.2, the sedentary life of the businessman (and perhaps woman now, as heart disease in women gains more attention; Healy 1991, Petticrew *et al.* 1993) was seen as a risk factor, as were the poor circumstances of the manual labourer. Individuals could therefore draw on a range of personal circumstances and social attributes to explain the observed pattern of illness in themselves, their families or wider communities.

This definite yet complex structure of lay epidemiology reveals an important issue which has a bearing on lay responses to health promotion campaigns as well as helping to understand the lack of fit between belief and behaviour noted by Pill *et al.* This is, to use Davison's phrase, that modes of explanation of illness are 'inherently fallible'. It has long been an argument of anthropologists that it is investigators rather than those investigated who strain towards seeing consistency in modes of thought, whether lay or professional,

Table 1.2 People who may be identified as coronary candidates

Fat people
People who don't take exercise and
are unfit
Red-faced people
People with a grey pallor
Smokers
People with heart trouble in the
family
Heavy drinkers
People who eat excessive amounts
of rich, fatty foods
Worriers (by nature)
Bad-tempered, pessimistic or
negative people

People who are under stress from	work
	family life
	financial difficulty
	unemployment/retirement
	bereavement
	gambling
People who suffer strain through	hard manual labour
	conditions of work/home
	over-indulgence (sex, dancing,
	drugs, lack of sleep, etc.)

Source: Davison *et al.* 1991: 13

common sense or scientific. Social actors, on the other hand, frequently demonstrate the ability to live with a degree of inconsistency or contradictoriness in belief (A. Young 1981) or perhaps more accurately, in the context of Davison's study, recognise ambiguity as being inherent even in a 'natural' event such as the onset of illness.

Lay experience testifies, for example, to the fact that many people suffer heart disease, and indeed die from it, without showing any clear evidence of behavioural or social risk factors, or where the combination of such factors provides a less than satisfactory answer to the question 'Why now?' This problem is likely to be ignored in population-based health promotion campaigns, in which everyone is told that they are at risk, though few may benefit (at least in terms of reduced mortality) from changing their lifestyles (Rose 1985). Lay observations provide frequent evidence of people who seem to have a range of 'risk factors' yet do not fall ill. It is the combination of these two contradictory processes (the presence of 'risk' but not its supposed correlates) that partly explains the inclusive character of the list of potential candidates given in Table 1.2. This also helps to explain, of course, that holding general beliefs about health risks does not necessarily lead to the adoption of specific health-promoting behaviours.

In an image which illustrates lay thinking in this area, Davison points to the existence of the apocryphal 'Uncle Norman' figure commonly talked about in the immediate or extended social networks of the sort found in South Wales and elsewhere (Davison *et al.* 1992: 682). Uncle Norman embodies (literally as well as metaphorically, perhaps) the problems that exist in linking indi-vidual experience and characteristics derived from the observations of populations. The Uncle Norman figure is overweight and red in the face, but 'survives into old age, despite extremely heavy smoking and drinking' (ibid.). The opposite kind of individual is also to be found in everyday life, slim and health conscious, but who may suffer the onset of disease or die a sudden death. Perhaps we might call her the 'Aunt Julia' figure.

This brings the discussion back to the earlier argument concerning the ambiguous nature of lay thinking about health and illness in changing societies, where fatalism can exist alongside explanatory frameworks. While scientific, abstract and expert systems have increasingly excluded notions of 'fortune' and 'fate' from everyday life, they may re-enter popular thought when profes-sional or expert systems fail in explanatory coverage or depth (Giddens 1991). Existential crises, especially those connected with the onset of serious illness – what Giddens calls 'disruptive moments' and what has been called, elsewhere in the medical soci-ology literature, 'biographical disruption' (Bury 1982) – create a need for a more complete form of explanatory thought. Fatalistic and perhaps religious ideas may be drawn upon to fill in the gaps that arise in official information and everyday observation.

In Davison's study, people reported several models which were able to deal with the element of the apparent randomness of some illnesses. One concerned a belief in the 'timely' nature of illness occurrence and of death; that is, the idea that people have an 'allotted' time, beyond which they are unlikely to live, no matter what their lifestyle may be. This echoes beliefs about death found in older people in Aberdeen (R. Williams 1990).

In an ironic vein, people in the South Wales study sometimes alluded to death (from a heart attack) in what Davison calls the 'pleasure boat setting', where the call rings out, 'Come in, number fourteen, your time is up!' In another image, war-time experiences were drawn upon, especially the random nature of bombing. This is based on the assumption that no amount of accurate prediction can ever say exactly where a bomb might end up falling, captured in the popular expression that 'if your number is on it' then you would 'catch it'. Such a notion is clearly capable of extension to disease onset, at least heart disease, in explaining the gap between lifestyle and the occurrence of illness.

Davison's study suggests, therefore, that lay beliefs are frequently a combination of ideas transmitted over time, and those derived from experience but then 'updated' in the light of official information circulating through the media and other sources, such as health promotion campaigns. This also suggests that in late modern cultures people are unlikely to show evidence of 'health beliefs' or a 'health belief system' that are sharply separate from official thinking. Indeed, it may well be that the latter itself draws on lay ideas in fashioning its own approach to health. Young has suggested as much in the field of stress (A. Young 1980), where lay ideas are reproduced in expert 'discourse' on the subject. People are seen, from this viewpoint, to be actively shaping their *beliefs and knowledge* under conditions of considerable social change. While moral dimensions are still evident in lay thinking about health and illness (Conrad 1994) these are constantly being exposed to both the certainties and inconsistencies in scientific and technical information. Shared ideas persist within stable communities, but are cut across by expert information.

CONCLUDING COMMENT

This chapter has charted the development of sociological research on 'lay' ideas, knowledge and behaviour with respect to health and illness. It has shown that in the 1970s medical sociologists concentrated mainly on illness-related behaviour and the use of, and encounters in, clinical health service settings. There will be more to say about changes on the latter topic in the discussion of the doctor–patient relationship (chapter 5). In more recent times, however, there has been a marked shift towards studying health beliefs and health behaviours in everyday settings, reflecting a cultural upsurge in attention to lifestyles and positive health. In addition, government policy and ideology has increasingly concentrated on emphasising individual responsibility for health.

Finally, the chapter has noted the tendency of sociological research to lend its support, sometimes unwittingly, to the pursuit of health promotion policies. Whilst this may be defended as assisting a move away from the earlier dominance of a 'mechanistic' medical model of health and illness, the emphasis on 'health and lifestyles' brings to the fore value problems of its own, especially that of individualism. The examples of work by Calnan and Davison were drawn upon here to indicate how this tension may be productively handled. They suggest that health beliefs and behaviour need to be set in the context of everyday life and the constraints which it involves, and not treated simply as individual attributes. If this is done, *lay knowledge* about health and illness can be explored more systematically. As the work of Davison in particular has shown, people have considerable knowledge about health and illness, derived from systematic observations made within specific communities. The idea that such knowledge should be treated as a matter of 'belief' runs the risk of underestimating the insights it can provide on the limitations of official views about health promotion. Such a view also suggests that health promotion activities should be based on an approach which can 'work with rather than against cultural norms and everyday principles of social organisation' as they relate to health (Backett and Davison 1995: 629). If this is done, the relevance of health promotion policies and the structure of lay views may both be approached positively in future sociological research.

Chapter 2

Inequalities in health

INTRODUCTION

During the same period as sociological interest in lay beliefs was developing, research and writing on inequalities in health was also growing apace, especially in Britain. Although this was influenced by the same social and political context as work on health beliefs, the tradition and style of research on inequalities has been quite different, and this has had important consequences. First, research on inequalities has been concerned with issues that relate more directly to the *public health* agenda and that of its scientific or academic discipline, *epidemiology*. Rather than studying the variability in the *meaning of health and illness*, as work on beliefs has inevitably done, those working in public health have traditionally been preoccupied with the social and geographical *distribution of disease*. As a result, emerging social research on inequalities has operated on the boundary between sociology and epidemiology, involving, at times, collaboration across disciplinary lines. Ironically, where conflict has broken out, at least in the academic debate, it has been among different sociological approaches rather than between sociology and public health medicine.

Part of the reason for this is that work on inequalities has relied heavily on the analysis of quantitative data, especially those derived from secondary sources such as mortality records and population censuses. The use of these official statistics has led to considerable controversy when used to display health inequalities. Though epidemiologists have usually been content with collecting, analysing and disseminating such data with a minimum of explanation, sociologists have been more concerned with establishing what their implications are, both theoretically and ideologically. The sociological controversy in this area has arisen because interpreting the evidence on health inequalities has to be derived from data that were not collected explicitly for the purpose – a classic example of what Catherine Marsh calls the problem with 'validity at the level of meaning'; where meaning is imported after the event (Marsh 1982). As result of this, and other factors to be discussed, the debate on inequalities in health has generated considerable heat, if not, at times, a proportionate amount of light.

In order to examine the issues at stake, the chapter proceeds along the following lines. First, the recent historical background and context of the debate is sketched in, including influences on the long-standing interest in health inequalities of public health specialists and the emerging concerns among sociologists. These developments are put in the context of the prevailing political and cultural climate in Britain, before and after 1945. Second, the chapter focuses on the evidence and argument presented with the publication of the Black Report in 1980 (Townsend and Davidson 1982), which remains one of the most influential documents on health inequalities, updated by Margaret Whitehead in 1990 with *The Health Divide* (Whitehead 1990, revised 1992).

Third, the chapter looks at the challenges and responses to the Black Report which emerged in the 1980s and have continued ever since. Finally, the chapter examines more recent sociological research which has attempted to move this debate forward. This offers the prospect of a more productive medical sociology research agenda on inequalities in the future. The policy and value implications of research on health inequalities are also returned to in this final section.

BACKGROUND AND CONTEXT TO THE INEQUALITIES DEBATE

The first thing that needs to be recognised in considering the inequalities debate is that there are considerable difficulties with the terms involved, especially the term 'inequalities' itself. This arises because the issues that are referred to are regarded as self-evident by some, but are challenged by others as highly problematic. To those in the first camp, the term 'inequalities' forms part of a general social critique that refers to the presence of structural deprivation and poverty, and to wealth and income differentials, not merely to natural 'differences' between people. There is little point, for example, in collecting detailed evidence about physical characteristics of individuals, say the colour of their eyes or hair, unless it has some relevance to life chances, including health. Evidence about the attributes of people only matters, to epidemiologists and sociologists at least, if they have *social* significance. It is, in the present context, the outcome of influences of *social position* on *health status* that matters, and invoking the term 'inequalities' frequently rests on the assumption that modern societies are characterised by *social hierarchies* (Mouzelis 1991) which structure and to some extent determine people's lives. A reduction in inequalities would mean lessening the impact of such hierarchies and thus creating a fairer society.

For others, however, the term 'inequalities' is problematic precisely because it conveys negative assumptions about social hierarchy which need to be examined. The main argument from this viewpoint is that those who use the term are really implying a value position, namely that they are *unacceptable*, and that a greater degree of equality should prevail. In contrast, it is held that inequalities are inevitable and even 'natural' features of all societies. Social inequalities (even marked ones) may also be justifiable, under modern conditions, on a number of grounds. In particular, it is suggested that social hierarchy needs to be seen as a function of *social mobility*, in that social divisions based on merit and hard work promote a social system which allows considerable social scope for personal advancement. Without inequalities the motivation to achieve would be weak because effort, it is held, would not receive its full reward. This position attempts to paint a more dynamic picture of social hierarchy and social divisions, drawing on a functionalist view of social stratification. Thus, inequalities from this point of view should not always be assumed to be unacceptable, as long as the differences between people are based on limited 'equity' in social life, including equal opportunities for personal advancement. If entrepreneurship and fair competition prevail (and especially where there is a general rise in the standard of living) the resulting differences between people may be seen as *acceptable inequalities*. Of course, a more recent conservative or 'neo-liberal' position is also implied here, and contrasts sharply with the 'left of centre' argument conveyed by many of the earlier proponents of the inequalities argument. And of course, there are many shades of opinion to be found in between these opposing views.

From the outset, then, the debate about health inequalities

involves fundamental ideological issues. When looked at from this viewpoint, it is perhaps understandable that controversy has characterised so much research on the subject. Perhaps it should be noted, however, that the health inequalities debate is not the only one to turn on the use of key terms where little agreement or consensus can be reached. Many areas of social life produce conflicts in attempts to control language. For example, terms such as 'peace', as in 'peace movements', and even 'life' itself, as in the 'pro life' campaigns, have become the focus of considerable social conflict. Moreover, controversy in Britain about academic approaches to broader dimensions of social inequalities, such as that which surrounded the launch of the educational initiative by the Open University with its course 'Patterns of Inequality' in the mid-1970s, suggested that any use of the term is likely to draw the fire of opponents, from one direction or another.

In fact, as Strong (1990a) and Vagero (1995) have pointed out, evidence and argument about inequalities and poverty, and the terms of the debate, are hardly new. Nor are actions to mitigate inequalities. Though Strong stretches the point, perhaps, by referring to welfare activity undertaken by the Roman Catholic Church in medieval times as a response to inequalities, as well as the proto welfare state in early modern Britain (Strong 1990a: 169), he rightly points to the importance of the systematic collection of information that has periodically characterised nearly every industrial society, certainly from the mid-eighteenth century onwards. At the least, the expansion of welfare systems was, from the outset, expensive, and has therefore involved the development of forms of 'social surveillance'. As a result, statistical techniques have become increasingly important to the governance of rapidly expanding populations and especially the development of urban living (Strong 1990a: 169).

In the first half of the twentieth century, public health campaigns were particularly vigorous, partly as the result of the adoption of an official classification of occupational class in 1911, which ranked occupations into five distinct groups and gave a new impetus to the collection of data along class lines (Strong 1990a: 170) and partly because of growing concerns with infant and maternal mortality. Political campaigns against poverty and what were known, during the slump of the 1930s, as the 'deprived areas' (Hannington 1937) were linked with these maternal and infant deaths. Indeed, arguments about death rates erupted throughout the 1930s, with public health campaigners blaming prevailing inequalities and poverty, and government supporters blaming feckless and irresponsible individuals. Debates about causes were, from an early date, routed through the newly expanding mass media, especially radio (Karpf 1988), and this gave a powerful new voice to critics of government policies, especially public health critics. As Vagero (1995) has pointed out, arguments about infant and maternal mortality were important in the setting up of modern welfare states in many European countries.

In the post-war period, however, the situation changed rapidly, especially with the new impetus behind the development of the modern welfare state, including, in Britain, the launch of the National Health Service (NHS) in 1948. Welfare and economic reconstruction seemed to overshadow the depression and deprivation of the 1930s. Living standards steadily rose and virtually full employment became a reality. The 'never had it so good' years of the 1950s and early 1960s were a time for optimism and, to some extent at least, for the development of a high degree of social consensus. As a result, the 'bitter memory of means testing' for welfare benefits during the 1930s faded (J.C. Brown 1994: 116). Few politicians of the right or the left offered any major criticism of the kind of economic planning that dominated post-war economies, or of the large-scale expansion of the welfare state, engineered by Beveridge. However, there were private expressions of doubt about the direction of British society and the mounting costs of welfare by leaders such as Macmillan as early as the 1950s (Hennessy 1996).

In the health field, the development of welfare and health services was accompanied by a gradual improvement in the health of the population, particularly in the reduction in infectious diseases among the young. Though there were epidemics of diseases such as whooping cough and poliomyelitis among children throughout the period up to the 1970s, these became increasingly rare. As the impact of the infections on early life lessened, so survival into middle and late life improved. This, together with the continuing decline in fertility rates, meant that countries such as Britain underwent a major 'demographic transition' towards an ageing population (Bury 1992a).

The implications of these improvements in 'the nation's health' for public health medicine were significant. The role that public health doctors had played, in between the two world wars, in drawing attention to the impact of poverty and deprivation on health appeared to wane. The growing importance of the acute medical sector, and the accompanying 'medical dominance' exercised by the hospital-based physicians and surgeons discussed in the first chapter of this book, had marginalised those working outside, including those working in public health and general practice. Though public health, with the academic discipline of epidemiology, became established in British medical schools during the post-war period and built on its ability to provide powerful statistical evidence of changing patterns of health and illness, its practical role in local authority health departments declined. As a result, it faced a considerable crisis of identity (Jefferys 1986). Criticisms of the inadequacy of a 'mechanistic' medical model and the lack of proper evaluation of many routine hospital procedures, made by public health specialists such as McKeown (1976) and Cochrane (1972) respectively, though attractive to sociologists working in the health field, were, in part, a reaction to this crisis, and served to underline the exclusion of public health doctors from the medical establishment.

However, throughout the 1960s a broader critique of post-war social and economic developments was developing from other quarters, especially a rapidly expanding sociology, and this provided common ground for co-operation with public health specialists. In what has sometimes been called the 'rediscovery of poverty' argument, sociologists challenged many of the assumptions that had underpinned the optimism of the post-war years (J.C. Brown 1994). In particular, it was argued, poverty had not been abolished and the pre-war class structure had survived post-war change, and continued to dominate British life (Wedderburn 1965; Westergaard and Resler 1976). Moreover, socialist and Marxist ideas underwent something of a revival in understanding modern Britain, albeit in their most familiar British disguise as Fabianism. In the mid-1960s Able Smith and Townsend produced *The Poor and the Poorest* (1965) and later Townsend went on to produce his compendious book *Poverty in the United Kingdom* (1979), which outlined and documented the argument that though living standards might have improved overall, the *relative* position of the poor had not improved in comparison with the wealthy. Major surveys of income and wealth distinction had already pointed in the same direction (Runciman 1966).

These general critiques of social inequalities were then extended and reinforced through the examination of health matters. Townsend had long had an interest in the welfare of groups such as the disabled and the elderly, and Able Smith had a particular interest in the Health Service. Links were forged in the 1960s between social scientists at the London School of Economics and the London School of Hygiene, where academic epidemiology had a strong and growing base. Sociologists were recruited into the School of Hygiene during the 1960s. As one of them, Margot Jefferys, has argued, the problems facing public health medicine – then called 'community medicine' – and its arguments with the medical establishment about the social and political dimensions of disease led it to find common cause with sociologists (Jefferys 1991). As indicated in chapter 1, many of the early posts in British medical sociology developed as a result of this growing co-operation.

The culmination of this renewed concern with inequalities in health occurred in April 1977, when the then Labour government set up the Working Group on Inequalities in Health under the chairmanship of Sir Douglas Black (then chief scientist at the Department of Health and later President of the Royal College of Physicians). The Group, which included Peter Townsend (at the time Professor of Sociology at Bristol), was asked to 'assemble available information' about social class and health to try to 'identify possible causal relationships' (Townsend and Davidson 1990: preface), as well as to make recommendations for future research. It is the report of this Working Group that has come to be known as the Black Report. When it was finally published, in 1980, the Labour government had been replaced by a Conservative administration under Margaret Thatcher, and the scene was set for a stormy launch.

The cultural and political climate had changed throughout the years in which the Working Group sat, and by the time it had finished the post-war consensus had all but disappeared. As a result, the report was inevitably treated with hostility by the new administration. Only 300 copies were published by the Department of Health, and strenuous efforts were made to play down the significance of its findings (Strong 1990a). The hostility to publishing data on inequalities, especially social class inequalities, has continued to this day, with sporadic skirmishes between statisticians and government ministers. Data on social class links with health and unemployment have been especially contentious in the publication of official statistics, including those produced for the annual report, *Social Trends* (Brindle 1995).

In order to understand the nature of the specific arguments

about the Black Report, two main steps need to be taken at this point. First, there is a need to provide a brief outline of the key findings of the report. Second, there is a need to examine the explanations and interpretations which were offered for them in the report and which have been the focus of so much of the subsequent discussion. The sections of the chapter that follow will concentrate largely on the analysis of occupational class differences, as these were the focus of the report. However, because of the growing importance of ethnicity and health throughout the period under consideration, this issue will also feature in the discussion. Gender differences have also received increasing attention during recent years and will be discussed as we proceed and underlined particularly in the final section of the chapter.

THE BLACK REPORT

There are many problems to be dealt with in examining the links between health and aspects of social structure such as class. The first is to define terms such as 'health' and 'class' in a way that makes them intelligible. The public health tradition has largely defined health by estimating disease levels and death rates. The first of these comprises measures of *morbidity* such as the number of new cases of disease occurring in a population within a given time period (disease 'incidence') or the number of cases of a particular disease present in a population at any given time (disease 'prevalence'). In recent times, under the influence of the demographic transition mentioned above, *disability* and *quality of life* measures have come to supplement the measurement of disease in estimating morbidity in older populations (Bowling 1995). In addition, estimates of hospital activity or the amount of 'sickness absence' may be used, though these are more a measure of illness behaviour than true morbidity.

Whilst recognising the importance of morbidity, however, the Black Report concentrates on marshalling and analysing data on *mortality.* Though more will be said later in the chapter about the decision to concentrate on this, the basic rationale given in the report is twofold. First, death rates provide relatively stable and thus comparable data *over time*, allowing comparisons between different groups of the population to be made, especially in the crucial period since 1945. Whilst using recorded deaths is not without its problems (for example, the rules or diagnostic conventions governing the recording of the causes of death may change), it does have the attraction of referring to a relatively clear-cut event, and is argued as being useful, therefore, 'mainly for practical reasons' (Townsend and Davidson 1990: 42).

Second, it is also argued that death rates provide an important, if sometimes crude, picture of the life chances of groups of people. In particular *premature death*, usually meaning deaths occurring under the age of 65, suggests that people may have died 'before their time', faintly echoing the biblical notion of an expectation of life of some 'three score years and ten'. By the same token, deaths in infancy have long been taken to be a particularly sensitive indicator of social conditions and the health of women in their child-bearing years.

For these reasons the Black Report focuses on death rates. Evidence on two measures of these will be summarised here. For adults, the Black Report bases much of its argument on the use of Standardised Mortality Ratios (SMRs): 'A method of comparing death rates between different sections of the population' (Townsend and Davidson 1990: 28). Specifically, this method provides a means of comparing the death rates of subgroups (e.g. particular social classes), standardised for age, with the rates for groups as a whole (e.g. for all men or women aged 15–64, in a given time period). By taking the average death rate for the whole group as 100, a ratio can be calculated which shows the actual experience of different social class groups compared with the expected average. For infants, the Black Report relies on Infant Mortality (IM) rates, which are calculated on the basis of the number of deaths occurring in the first year of life per thousand live births (excluding stillbirths and deaths that occur at or around the time of death – so-called 'perinatal' mortality). As will be seen, recent debates about ethnicity and health inequalities have also relied on infant mortality data.

Mention has already been made of the origins and development of the other major category to be used here, social class. In Britain at least, gathering routine information on occupational groups began in the early 1900s through the use of the Registrar General's Classification of Occupations. Despite its widespread use, this scheme has attracted considerable criticism over the years, especially from feminists, for its male bias and for the way women have been classified by their husband's occupation (Arber 1990). This issue will be returned to at the end of the chapter. However, its use is defended in the Black Report for pragmatic reasons, namely that official data on deaths by occupational groups have been collected over long periods of time using the scheme, allowing for trends to be examined. The Black Report summarises the occupational categories used in the classification in the following manner:

I   Professional (e.g. accountant, doctor, lawyer)
II   Intermediate (e.g. manager, nurse, schoolteacher)
IIINM   Skilled non-manual (clerical worker, secretary, shop assistant)
IIIM   Skilled manual (e.g. bus driver, carpenter, coal-face worker)
IV   Partly skilled (e.g. agricultural worker, bus conductor, postman)
V   Unskilled (e.g. cleaner, dock worker, labourer)

(Townsend and Davidson 1990: 40)

Having clarified the main dependent variable, mortality, and the main independent variable, social class, the discussion can now proceed to summarise the main findings of the Black Report. As Figure 2.1 shows, in the case of adults between the ages of 15 and 64, for virtually all causes of death there is a consistent *inverse relationship between social class and mortality*. That is, the higher the social class group, the lower its SMR, and conversely the lower the social class group, the higher its SMR. The most marked SMR gradient shown in Figure 2.1 occurs in the case of respiratory disorders in men, though it is present in nearly every other category, irrespective of gender. The exceptions shown are 'malignant neoplasm' (cancer) and accidents, violence and poisoning in women.

Though the report makes it clear that death rates in general for this age group have improved (that is, they have fallen) over time, when SMRs are calculated they show that the *relative* position of social class groups has remained remarkably stable. So while mortality has been improving for the population as a whole, the gap between social class groupings has remained wide. This implies that people from 'higher' occupational groups have maintained their favourable position even though improvements have occurred throughout the population as a whole. Indeed, more recent evidence has tended to suggest, in support of the Black Report, that data for the years 1979–83 compared with those for 1970–2 (as shown in Figure 2.1 from the Black Report) show a worsening in the position of social class V, from an SMR of 137 to 165 for all causes of

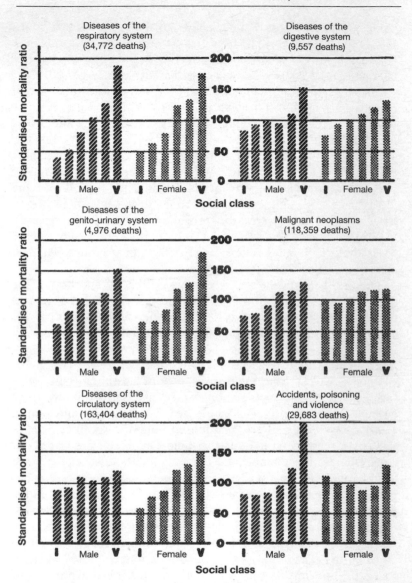

Figure 2.1 Occupational class and mortality in adult life (men and married women 15–64) by husband's occupation 1970–72

Source: Townsend and Davidson 1990: 47. Crown copyright is reproduced with the permission of the Controller of HMSO.

death. Remembering that the average for SMRs is 100, this means that social class V changed from being 37 to 65 points worse than the average. Social class I improved from an SMR of 77 to one of 66, that is, from 23 to 34 points better than the average (*BMJ* 1986).

As far as adult mortality and ethnicity is concerned, the picture is not as straightforward as social class, if only because of additional difficulties in defining ethnic status, across generations and between groups. In addition, immigration makes estimates difficult, as base-line populations may undergo rapid change within short periods of time (e.g. the arrival of refugees following war). Though population censuses carried out in Britain have not allowed the identification of ethnic minorities, change in the collection of data from the 1991 census onwards, providing details of ethnic status, will help to tackle this problem. Data are already revealing higher levels of long-standing illness in minority ethnic groups (Dunnel, cited in Smaje 1995: 44).

Despite the difficulties in researching ethnicity and health, the *Health Divide* which, it will be remembered, provided a revised update of the Black Report in 1992 (Whitehead 1992), does provide a summary of the main findings of the Immigrant Mortality Survey (Marmot *et al.* 1984). Some of the most important of these are given in Table 2.1.

Table 2.1 shows that for many causes of death, mortality rates for immigrants are considerably worse in comparison with the average for the country as a whole (see also Balarajan and Bulusu 1990). However, the inverse relationship found in social class analysis is not reproduced in quite the same way. Men from Caribbean backgrounds, for example, have lower SMRs than the average (Smaje 1995: 36). This suggests that ethnic minority status does not predict health status in any simple manner. This is discussed in the Black Report, with respect to data which show that ethnic minorities classified in the upper occupational groups have considerably better SMRs than those in 'lower' occupational groups (Townsend and Davidson 1990: 51). The issue of the interaction of different variables in inequalities research will be returned to at the end of this chapter.

Turning to *infant mortality*, first in general terms, the Black Report suggests that variations in experience by social class mirror those found in adult mortality. It states that:

Table 2.1   Summary of the Immigrant Mortality Study (England and Wales) 1970–78

Mortality by cause	Comparison with death rates for England and Wales
Tuberculosis	*High* for immigrants from India, Indian sub-continent, Ireland, Caribbean, Africa, Scotland
Cancer of stomach, large intestine, breast	*Low* among Indians
Ischaemic heart disease	*High* mortality in immigrants from Indian sub-continent
Violence and accidents	*High* in all immigrant groups

Source: Adapted from Whitehead 1992: 258

For the death of every one male infant of professional parents, we can expect almost two among children of skilled manual workers and three among children of unskilled manual workers. Among females the ratios are even greater.

(Townsend and Davidson 1990: 44)

Here it needs to be remembered that these findings are of the *relative position* of infants from different occupational classes. Overall, in the period up to the time of the Black Report, infant mortality rates had fallen to an historic low, and in 1996 stood at some 7 per 1000 live births. It is the relationship between infants of parents from different class backgrounds that the report highlights, reinforcing its argument that though indicators such as infant mortality have changed for the better in absolute terms, poorer groups have still not closed the gap with the better off.

However, if the relationship between infant mortality and ethnic status is considered, this again presents a more complex story. Whitehead, summarising data from a later report from the Office of Population Censuses and Surveys (OPCS), shows that infant mortality among minority ethnic groups from Irish, Bangladeshi or Indian countries of origin is comparable with that of groups from UK backgrounds, but those from Pakistan and the Caribbean have markedly worse rates, approximately 14 per 1000 live births, twice that of the UK as a whole. Whitehead makes the point, however, that the Pakistani and Caribbean groups, among ethnic minorities, are the only ones to 'show excess mortality throughout infancy' (Whitehead 1992: 260). Drawing on similar data, a later report by Andrews and Jewson (1993) shows that mothers from Pakistan and the Caribbean experience an infant mortality rate of 16 per 1000. Higher rates are found when other forms of mortality are brought into the picture, for example perinatal and neonatal deaths. Diversity in minority ethnic experience is combined with instances of high death rates for some groups.

In sum, the Black Report has provided evidence of a persistent class gradient in mortality, despite the improvements experienced by all groups in the post-war period. Mirroring the 'rediscovery of poverty' argument developed in mainstream sociology, data from the health field have seemed to confirm the contention, long held by such commentators, that the capitalist system has not only kept the poor in their place but has also meant that they have shorter lives and experience worse health among their offspring. Despite (or, perhaps, because of) this strongly argued case, criticism and counter-argument broke out as soon as the Black Report was published. However, it is not so much the evidence that has been challenged, but the explanations given for it. These are now summarised in the next section.

EXPLANATIONS FOR INEQUALITIES IN HEALTH

Although the public health experts and sociologists on the Working Group that produced the Black Report went to considerable lengths to marshal evidence on health inequalities, the 'crunch' of the report came in trying to explain them. It is one thing to show that the poor have worse health and die younger than the rich, and that some deprived ethnic minorities fare badly, but another to say why. It will be remembered that the Working Group's remit included the consideration of possible *causal* relationships involved in linking data on health with social factors, a much more difficult problem to tackle.

The Conservative government that issued the report in 1980 was quick to state, in the words of the health minister at the time, Patrick Jenkin, 'It is disappointing that the Group were unable to make greater progress in disentangling the various causes of inequalities in health' (Townsend and Davidson 1990: foreword).

Though this may well have been a way of avoiding the main thrust of the report – the inverse relationship between class and health described above – there is little doubt that deriving statements of cause from such findings is a complex issue. The Black Report's own approach was to summarise four main 'theoretical' lines of explanation under the following headings: artefact explanations, social selection, cultural and behavioural explanations and materialist or structuralist explanations. In what follows the main points of these approaches and some of the evidence for considering them are summarised, before the chapter goes on to discuss the different positions that have been taken up in the subsequent debate.

Artefact explanations

This explanation of observed health inequalities 'suggests that both health and class are artificial variables' (Townsend and Davidson 1990: 105) and that, therefore, trying to derive causal relationships is a false exercise. Here, in contrast to the idea that statistics can speak for themselves, it is suggested that they can be made to fit an author's case, and are therefore unreliable as a basis for sound causal inferences. We have already noted the difficulty of using routine statistics in this context. The alleged artificiality of the variables under consideration in part arises from the fact that social and cultural change has considerably affected their 'construction' over time. Two main points have been made in this connection.

First, the uses of mortality statistics as a measure of health, especially for adults under the age of 65, may be misleading at a time when steady improvements in survival have occurred. Showing the *relative* position of social class groupings (through the use of SMRs, for example) for ages 16–64, as remaining the same between different historical periods, disguises the fact that the proportion of deaths occurring in this age group has decreased steadily in the post-war period. Death now occurs much more frequently in old age, as the earlier comments on the 'demographic transition' suggested. Illsley, for example, has pointed out that 'In 1921 only 32% of males died at 65 or later; by 1971 it was 65%' (Illsley 1987: 16). In other words, the picture presented by comparing SMRs over time, among adults, does not show that figures increasingly refer to an ever smaller proportion of deaths.

Second, the social class composition of countries such as Britain has also undergone rapid change, as the economy has been restructured and drawn into 'globalising' processes. This has had the effect of reducing the proportion of the population in many working-class occupations and expanding the service industries. For example, in 1951 there were 766,000 people working in the coal industry and 571,000 in metal manufacture; by 1991 these numbers had fallen to 80,000 and 166,000 respectively (Law 1994: 92). Overall employment in the industrial sector had fallen from 9.4 million in 1951 to just over 5 million in 1991 (ibid.). Concomitantly, we find that in 1951 some 10.5 million people worked in the service sector, and by 1991 this figure had risen to over 15.5 million (Law 1994: 93) with an important increase in the proportion comprising women. When these changes are taken into account, it may be additionally misleading to present the mortality of occupational groups without showing how such groups have changed from one historical period to another. The proportion of the working population in 'higher' occupational groups (with their more favourable survival pattern) has expanded.

Social selection

Linked to the above points, the social selection explanation suggests that change in both health status and social class over time makes the *causal direction* of any argument about them difficult to disentangle. For *cause* to be demonstrated, the temporal sequence of events has to be established, as well as co-variance between variables (de Vauss 1990: 5, 41).

In the case of class and health, the main line of the Black Report is that the causal direction is from the former to the latter: that is, that a person's class position influences their health status. However, theoretically the relationship could be the other way round, namely that poor health has an impact on class formation and position. Poor health may cause a 'drift' down the occupational ladder, and therefore influence a person's class position. The possibility of this being a significant explanation for health inequalities is not new, especially in the mental health field, where it has long been argued that serious mental illness may lead to 'social drift' (Hollingshead and Redlich 1958). As people move between social and class groupings – that is, where they live in a society with a given level of *social mobility* – it cannot be ruled out that health status (together with other characteristics) influences a person's life chances and therefore their social class. More will be said about this argument below.

Cultural/behavioural explanations

Under this heading, the issues of lifestyle, choice and individual responsibility for health, discussed in chapter 1 in the context of health beliefs, enter the inequalities debate. In the somewhat loaded terms of the Black Report, these kinds of explanation 'often focus on the individual as a unit of analysis emphasizing unthinking reckless or irresponsible behaviour or incautious life-style as the moving determinant of poor health' (Townsend and Davidson 1990: 110). However, though this suggests that cultural explanations lead to forms of individualistic 'victim blaming' for health (Crawford 1977) the report does go on to show that some health behaviours vary significantly by social class.

The most obvious example is smoking. It will be remembered that the steepest gradient for SMRs between the social classes (see Figure 2.1) was that for respiratory illness and malignant neoplasm. One explanation for part of the additional burden experienced by working-class groups is the disproportionate smoking rates in these groups, as shown in Table 2.2.

The step-wise relationship between class and smoking is striking. This is especially relevant to claims that 80 per cent of cases of lung cancer, in particular, are caused by smoking (Standing Medical Advisory Committee 1994). As was argued in chapter 1, sociologists

Table 2.2   Cigarette smoking by socio-economic group (males and females aged 16+) 1992

SEG	Current smokers %	
	Men	Women
Professional	14	13
Managerial	23	21
Intermediate NM	25	27
Skilled M	34	27
Semi-skilled M	39	31
Unskilled M	42	35
All	29	28

Source: CSO 1995

are keen to contextualise such data, not only in cultural terms but also in relation to the constraints of the environment. This includes such issues as the effects of poverty and stress, as Hilary Graham's work on smoking and women shows (Graham 1987, 1993), where structural influences on the link between behaviour and health status are made evident.

Of course, smoking is not the only example where this kind of explanation is relevant, and other forms of 'risk' behaviours such as alcohol consumption, diet and exercise have also received consider-able attention. Whilst the Black Report recognises that health behaviours are significant, it resists placing too much emphasis on them. This is partly because overemphasis on them reinforces an individualistic level of analysis, but also because they bolster the ideological interests of dominant groups, for whom a recognition of the effects of social structures is anathema.

The report quotes, in this connection, the words of Edwina Currie, minister of health in Britain in 1986 : 'I honestly don't think that it [the link between deprivation and health] has anything to do with poverty. The problem very often for many people is just igno-rance . . . and failing to realise that they do have some control over their lives' (Townsend and Davidson 1990: 12). At the time, this statement seemed to represent the official position on health and risk behaviour, namely that if culture and behaviour were discussed, they quickly boiled down to a charge of 'ignorance'. Though, socio-logically, it is important to recognise that people are not merely passive victims of circumstance or 'social context', it has already been indicated that there is little evidence of widespread ignorance of official health information. And, for sociologists, culture refers to 'deep rooted patterns of ideas and values which are often trans-mitted from one generation to the next, and as such represent long term influences on human behaviour' (Vagero and Illsley 1995: 221). This is despite the fact that people may make choices which trade off health for other valued goals. The difficulties in developing cultural and behavioural explanations are, however, underlined by these considerations.

Materialist/structuralist explanations

Materialist explanations direct attention to aspects of the social structure, especially deprivation and poverty, that arguably have direct or indirect consequences for health. As will be clear by now, it is to these 'strands of reasoning' (Townsend and Davidson 1990: 106) that the report, its findings and recommendations are essentially addressed. However, the report recognises that, in the political context referred to above, appeals to 'material inequality' in the sense of the *direct* effects of 'exploitation and poverty' may be considered of only historical interest, associated with 'the urban slums of Victorian and Edwardian cities' or the 'shanty towns of the underdeveloped world' in our own times (ibid.). After all, many people today, including working-class people, have consumer goods and holidays (including foreign holidays), unheard of in previous times (Obelkevich and Catterall 1994: 5).

The Black Report attempts to challenge these assumptions by developing two lines of argument. First, it states that 'basic needs', in the sense of being able to meet *physiological* requirements, may still be a problem for many people in countries such as Britain, implying that some elements of absolute poverty still exist. The ability to provide food, clothing and housing in order to sustain life is presumably what is meant here, though Sen (1984) includes a basic level of self-esteem in his definition (see also Vagero and Illsley 1995 on this point). Second, a more relative view of poverty is invoked, which may lead to disadvantage in work and 'social obligations' and which may go on to have an effect on risk of illness or accident or on 'the factors actively promoting health' (Townsend and Davidson 1990: 107).

The report documents a number of the strands that go to make up relative poverty. These include the effects of new industrial processes on the lives of working people and on the communities and environments in which they are located; income disparities, in being above or below officially designated supplementary levels; and unemployment and recession, which weaken 'supportive relationships and networks, and in general, a more varied and more elevated meaning for human existence' (Townsend and Davidson 1990: 110). The report's main recommendations for tackling child poverty, the allocation of health resources on the basis of need (as measured, in part, by SMRs) and greater emphasis on prevention and care in the community, flow from this approach.

Thus, in the Black Report, the notion of 'materialist or structuralist' explanations for health inequalities covers a wide range of factors. These range from the direct effects of poverty and low income to the admittedly more vague aspects of stress and community-level hardship that may flow from them (Vagero and Illsley

1995). Such material factors may also produce a subjective sense of disadvantage, as people become increasingly aware of inequalities between different social groups within an aggressive consumer culture. On this latter point it is the social distribution of rewards and status that matters, rather than poverty alone.

However, this approach to the different elements of a materialist explanation is both its strength and its weakness. On the one hand it directs attention to important features of the social structure and how they might singly, or in combination, be causally implicated in health disorders. On the other hand, the widening of 'materialist/ structuralist' explanations to cover aspects of meaning, such as the experience of stress and breakdown in social relationships and a sense of status disparity, creates a potentially unwieldy analytic device. The tensions between these various factors, between absolute and relative poverty and between poverty and inequality, together with the different levels of analysis they imply, help explain why the Black Report has become the focus of considerable debate in the fifteen years or so since it was published.

CHALLENGES AND RESPONSES TO THE BLACK REPORT

Of all the challenges issued by medical sociologists to the Black Report, that of Raymond Illsley, already mentioned, is perhaps the most important. Though Illsley has not disputed the accuracy of the data shown in the report, he has mounted a sustained assault on the explanations for them, especially the emphasis on materialist factors. In contrast to the report's approach, he has sought to clarify the significance of some of the key changes in both health and class discussed in the previous section. Though Illsley has published several accounts of his objections to the Black Report's argument (Illsley 1980, 1986; Illsley and Baker 1991; Illsley and Le Grand 1987) his paper in the *Quarterly Journal of Social Affairs* provides us with an exposition of his main points (Illsley 1986, but see also Stern 1983).

The first point Illsley develops concerns both the artefact and social selection explanations for observed inequalities. Illsley questions the scientific validity of comparing death rates of occupational classes over long periods of time because of important changes in the definitions and boundaries of such classes. The Black Report, Illsley suggests, treats social class as a being 'reified as if it had a physical existence', and asks what it can mean to compare 'Class V in 1931 and in 1971' (Illsley 1986: 152). In fact, during this period Class I 'increased from 1.8% of the economically active male population to 5%... while Class V fell from 12.9% to 8.4%' (Illsley 1986: 153).

Though it might be objected that Durkheimian sociology has always suggested that 'social facts should be treated as things' and that some degree of 'reification' is always involved in developing second-order constructs, Illsley's point is that the problems with social class analysis are particularly acute when seen in the context of 'selective change' in society. Illsley states: 'If a decreasing Class V is becoming more and more negatively selective and if an increasing Class I is selecting positively from lower groups', then by definition 'classes with high death rates now form a much smaller segment of our society, and classes with low rates a much larger segment' (Illsley 1986: 155). Though it is still possible to argue about the significance of this trend for understanding health inequalities, there is little doubt that the 'character of classes has been massively affected by changes in the absolute and relative size of occupational classes' (Illsley 1986: 156). When this is taken into account a class analysis of the sort offered by the Black Report, with its emphasis on marked and persistent differences between apparently stable groups, appears difficult to sustain.

Second, Illsley argues that the selection processes alluded to in his objection to the report can be examined by drawing on a large-scale data set from the Aberdeen Maternity and Neonatal Bank, which covers the period 1951–80 (Illsley 1986: 158). The level of social mobility shown in these data across the time period concerned, Illsley argues, is similar to that shown in other, more general studies of social mobility, notably that of Goldthorpe et al. (1980). More important from the viewpoint of health inequalities is that the data appear to show clear evidence of health playing a part in the selective process.

By comparing the social class position of women during their 'upbringing' with that of their 'class at marriage' (that is, ascribed versus achieved class) Illsley shows that health variables, for example low birth weight and height, in combination with social factors such as educational level, correlate well with movement either up or down the social class scale. The assumption in the Black Report of an unchanging or even increasing gap between the social classes is held to be untenable in the face of such selective processes. If these are taken into account 'it is possible to envisage

the occupational class gap as an inevitable consequence of occupational mobility and of selective class recruitment and loss' (Illsley
1986: 162).

Illsley concludes his argument with the assertion that 'concentra-
tion upon class rates and differences has diverted attention away
from the striking heterogeneity existing within classes' (Illsley 1986:
164). It might also be added that Illsley's argument implies that
reliance in the Black Report on 'snapshots' of class death rates at
different points, through the use of an SMR 'grid', is bound to
produce a similar picture at different points in time, no matter what
changes have taken place to the absolute and relative sizes of the
groups underneath. Because of this the report's approach to
inequalities also fails to shed light on the magnitude of broader
social and cultural change across the time periods concerned. It also
disguises the fact that the period that the report relies on, namely
the 1970s, was actually the culmination of a long period of
'decreasing income inequality', though this was reversed in the
1980s (Vagero and Illsley 1995: 225).

However, given the thrust of Illsley's criticisms, responses by
those supporting the Black Report were not long in appearing. In
particular Wilkinson (1986), Blane et al. (1993), Davey Smith et al.
(1990, 1991, 1994) and Whitehead, in her *Health Divide* update of
the Black Report (Whitehead 1992), are of note here. Two main
points may be taken from these counter-arguments.

First, they suggest that in analysing factors that may affect social
mobility intergenerationally, as we have seen Illsley does, the relative
weight of health versus non-health factors needs to be assessed.
These authors argue that studies of social mobility, such as that of
Goldthorpe et al. (1980), actually show that the major determinants
'are education and the material and cultural backgrounds of the
family, rather than health' (Whitehead 1992: 313). Second, Blane et
al. (1993) argue that the mobility between classes found in Illsley's
study mostly took place between classes III, IV and V. Movement
between classes close to each other, and for reasons other than
health, suggests that the scale of the 'massive effects' of social class
change may be less than Illsley thinks.

But Illsley has not been the only critic of the Black Report.
Other, and to some extent, sharper views followed Illsley's assault.
Illustrative of the tenor of some of the debate is a series of
exchanges which followed the publication of a pamphlet with the
title *Acceptable Inequalities?* by the right-wing 'think tank', the

Institute of Economic Affairs (Green 1988). Here the ideological basis of the Black Report and its argument are given greater attention. In the pamphlet, Klein in particular reiterated many of the criticisms made by Illsley, including the difficulties in assessing the stability of social class groups over time, the problems of relying on data from the working population in an ageing society, and selective mobility. On the last point Klein claimed that 'the Black Report brushes aside the evidence that at least some of the differences between the social classes reflect selective social mobility' (Klein 1988: 11). Though Klein nails his colours to the mast of reducing inequalities, which, he says, in an extreme form 'like the worst kinds of pornography, corrupt the sensibilities of society' (Klein 1988: 4), he castigates those who regard any challenge to the Black Report as a form of 'betrayal' (Klein 1988:10).

Subsequently, a series of articles appeared in the *International Journal of Health Services* in which Townsend and Klein traded several punches. Townsend's defence of the Black Report against Klein (and thus Illsley) can be summarised briefly, as many of the main points have already been made. First, as far as social class is concerned, Townsend argues that Klein fails to take account of much of the work following Illsley's critique, showing that by careful analysis of social class groupings, especially combining class I and II and class IV and V, much of the importance of the growth in class I and decline in class V is reduced. Townsend states that, in considering present class inequalities, 'while there are problems of operational measurement, and undoubted problems in pinning down the trend for each sex, there can be no scientific doubt about the direction of the trend' (Townsend 1990: 367).

Second, in reply to Klein's point about the reliance on data from people of working age, Townsend cites more recent work carried out by the OPCS. An analysis of class mortality across a wider age range by Fox *et al.* (1986) found that differentials persisted throughout later life. Even at age 85, the authors argue, a marked class gradient in mortality can be seen, implying as others have suggested that labour market position has implications for life chances through and into retirement and beyond (Walker 1981).

Third, as far as the social selection hypothesis is concerned, Townsend accepts that linking health with social mobility is necessary 'in providing a total explanation of inequalities in health' (Townsend 1990: 368). However, he reiterates the Black Report's position that having recognised the complexities involved, 'we wish to stress the importance of differences in material conditions of life' (Townsend 1990: 369). In support of this, Townsend mentions further studies 'on unemployment and suicide and for specific occupations' which weaken 'the likely causal contribution made by social mobility' (ibid.).

In reply, Klein (1991) attempts again to move the debate away from arguments about the data and methodology and to 'deconstruct' what he regards as the emotional responses to the Black Report, which has become an 'intellectual icon' (Klein 1991:175). Developing his argument, Klein states that if 'the Black Report arouses passion it is because it is essentially part of a political programme'. Klein's own approach (arguably no less political, of course) is to ask 'whether health policy should be exclusively driven by a concern about inequality . . . or whether maximising the population's health should be an equally desirable policy objective' (ibid.). Here Klein reflects the changing political climate of the 1980s, mentioned at the beginning of this chapter, in which inequalities may be acceptable, even desirable, if they are part of an economic and social dynamic which offers general improvements and wide opportunity to the population as a whole. Social inequalities should therefore be examined critically, rather than be assumed, *a priori*, to be wrong. The Black Report and those supporting it, according to Klein, fail to scrutinise the premises on which it is based.

Klein concludes that though the Black Report has revitalised the debate on health inequalities, the emphasis on persistent class differences overdramatises and at the same time simplifies the issues. This, Klein argues, provides 'an excuse for inaction by policy makers' (Klein 1991: 181) and avoids the need for a deeper understanding. Though Townsend subsequently replied to Klein's attack (Townsend 1991) this added little that was new, and largely confined itself to the argument that critics such as Klein were simply ignoring the evidence for and the significance of persistent inequalities.

Despite this intellectual stalemate the debate on health inequalities can still be regarded as one of the most important to have occurred in British medical sociology in the last fifteen years. The collaboration of sociologists and public health epidemiologists, who had earlier dominated the analysis of health trends, is notable. The Black Report has clearly provided an important focus for this debate ('intellectual icon' may be stretching a point) and for those who have sought to develop further aspects of the issue. The most recent comparative work by Wilkinson on income and health (Wilkinson 1992, 1994), which shows that infant mortality is lower in countries with a more equal distribution of income (though see Judge 1995 for a critique), and Bartley (1994) on the direct and indirect effects of unemployment, are cases in point. In addition, in 1994 the British government set up a Standing Committee within the Department of Health to monitor health inequalities and to commission new research, and in 1995 the King's Fund published a report on the policy implications of health inequalities (Benzeval *et al.* 1995). In late 1995 a further research initiative on 'health variations' (the preferred term in official circles) was also launched by the Economic and Social Research Council. This to some extent illustrates the impact that the health inequalities debate continues to have at the policy and research levels, Klein's criticisms notwithstanding.

Having said this, it might also be argued that the Black Report's approach and its legacy can be seen in a more pessimistic light. The suggestion throughout the debate is not only that class differences have worsened over time but also that ethnic minorities fare badly, in addition to persistent poverty among such groups as the elderly and disabled. Women's health is also increasingly seen as a problem area requiring similar documentation (Doyal 1996). This view conveys the idea that little improvement in health has occurred in the post-war period, and is unlikely to in future without a major redistribution of income and wealth. Given the political direction of most, if not all, industrialised countries, this seems to give some credence to one of Klein's charges, namely that the debate produces a sense of powerlessness in the face of massive disadvantage and an inability to alter its course. Couched in these terms, the health inequalities debate has sometimes threatened to become a sterile one.

Indeed, the positive role of *social action* (what might be called the agency question) in the field of health inequalities is all but absent in the debate. The emphasis on material and structural factors all too readily creates a picture of 'the poor', 'the working class' or 'ethnic minorities' as victims of circumstance. To this extent critics such as Illsley and Klein make an important point, namely that there is a danger in overemphasising structural factors, of not recognising change and improvement when they have occurred and of failing to explore the benefits which expanding health services have brought about. Ironically it is Sir Douglas

Black who has recently drawn attention to evidence on the contribution medical care can make to public health, including reducing mortality rates in the case of diseases 'amenable to treatment' (Black 1994). Vagero also has an important point in stressing the need to address positive and specific public health policies, in areas which 'give most cause for concern' (Vagero 1995: 14). Targeting death rates from cancer, for example, or infant mortality (both over-represented in poorer groups) might be a means of reconciling reducing inequalities and tackling the health of the poor, with improving health at a broader level (Vagero 1995). This might act as a focus for collective action, when radical redistributionist policies are unrealistic.

Without such a perspective, there is also the possibility that reductions in health provision may be encouraged by health inequality arguments, which point to the apparent inability of welfare states to effect positive change. There seems little point in defending collectivist health and welfare systems if they have little beneficial effects on inequalities. Having said this, some medical sociologists have recently been developing new and fresh lines of research, which have attempted to overcome some of these difficulties. These have addressed, in particular, the important question of social and cultural change which has dogged the heels of the health inequalities debate. A brief résumé of some of this more recent work can therefore act as an appropriate conclusion to the chapter.

CONCLUDING COMMENTS

In considering the future directions in the inequalities debate a number of points can be made. First, and in an implicit reply to Klein's call for a 'deeper understanding' of the issues involved, Macintyre (1986, 1994) has offered a detailed analysis of the 'social patterning' of health, incorporating factors such as class, ethnicity, gender and regional variations. These factors, she has argued, can variously affect a person's 'social position' and hence health. Such an approach not only has the benefit of moving away from a reliance on one factor such as social class, but also helps cope with the scale of social change that has occurred in modern communities. For example, Macintyre shows that risk of high mortality may be associated with being resident in a high-risk locality, but reduced by living in a better-off part of it (Macintyre 1994: 55). Moreover, citing Williams' work (R. Williams 1993) Macintyre makes the point that regional patterns have changed significantly over time, reflecting the pattern of industrialisation and associated factors (see also R. Williams 1994).

Through using data from a longitudinal study in Glasgow (the '20-07' study) Macintyre and her colleagues have attempted to unravel some of the complexities of the links between social structure and ill health in a changing environment. In particular, they have addressed the reliance on importing 'material factors' after the event, and on a rather crude use of marital status ('men and married women') in work exemplified by the Black Report.

In the 20-07 study, a number of indicators of social position are used in addition to occupation, for example home occupancy and the ownership of consumer goods such as cars. The latter may stand as a measure for 'material resources' where direct information on matters such as income may be unreliable (Wyke and Ford 1992: 526). This is in line with work being developed elsewhere. Davey Smith *et al.* (1991), for example, also cite the use of car ownership in a longitudinal study carried out by the OPCS, which also addresses the need for 'indices of socio-economic position other than social class' (Davey Smith *et al.* 1991: 351). The roles of social support and marital status are also taken into account in the 20-07 study, as are objective and subjective assessments of health. This aims to provide a more fine-grained picture, both of the variables that influence health status and of the definition of health itself. One of the main findings of the survey has been to suggest that 'no longer married men and women fared worse on almost every health measure compared to married men and women' and were most likely to have few material resources (Wyke and Ford 1992: 530). In this way the immediate context of household environments and material factors are being brought together in a more satisfactory manner. The 'complex picture' called for by Klein is now being constructed, providing an important window not only on health but also on key features of contemporary social experience.

One of the most important of these is, of course, changes in the social and economic position of women. Throughout the debate on inequalities, gender differences have often been noted, but not examined systematically. This is now changing with the work of sociologists such as Arber drawing attention to the interaction between the structural position of women (where occupation is assessed independently of male partners) and the impact of gender roles on health (Arber 1990). Arber has also gone on to explore the gendered patterning of health in later life (Arber and Ginn 1991), arguing that age and gender should feature more prominently in feminist and medical sociology (Arber 1994). Social epidemiologists are also exploring the nature of processes such as 'blocked' social mobility – the so-called 'glass ceiling' problem – in women and its impact on health (Roberts *et al.* 1993).

Second, in addition to new approaches to social patterning, the element of 'agency' is also being explored more systematically, and this too is showing the potential for unravelling some of the knots tied up in the Black Report. For example, as discussed in chapter 1, the links between health behaviour, gender and social class, within a culture increasingly dominated by health promotion messages, have been analysed by Calnan and his colleagues (Calnan 1987). In this work, cultural and behavioural explanations for health are seen to relate closely to *hierarchical* social relations, and not simply individual 'attitudes' or 'attributes' (see chapter 1). Lifestyle choices are thus being examined as actions fashioned within specific everyday contexts. As with Arber, this work also has the benefit of drawing attention to inequalities in health other than those linked to mortality data.

Similarly, Blaxter's work on *Health and Lifestyles* has pointed to the ways in which contextualising health behaviours can help explain risk behaviours (Blaxter 1990). Importantly, Blaxter's work has suggested that one of the reasons for the greater attachments to some forms of risk behaviour in working-class life is that the experience of health gains from adopting 'healthier' lifestyles may be greater in more middle-class groups. Risk behaviour may not always show a consistent pattern and the benefits of a healthier lifestyle (in terms of morbidity and subjective health status) are seen more readily among those who live and work in a healthier environment (Blaxter 1990: 221). In this way the *meanings* attached to health and the context in which these are fashioned are brought into much-needed focus.

However, in later discussions Blaxter has also gone on to emphasise the importance that *time* has in explaining why, despite all the arguments about the Black Report, 'the poor' themselves rarely refer to material or structural settings in interviews about their health (Blaxter 1992, 1993). Though the Black Report may show consistent data on mortality inequalities over time, from an *experiential* viewpoint or at the level of *meaning* this is rarely the case. As was shown in chapter 1, when people compare their own health with that of their parents they consistently report substantial change for the better. Blaxter's point, as in Macintyre's work, is that unless the temporal element is explored with respect to active involvement in changing communities, the inequalities debate is likely to make little contact with the sociological realities of late modern cultures. This may be especially true in a period of 'disorganised capitalism', marked by changing class structures and by the undermining of local and regional economies by a process of 'globalisation' involving considerable cultural complexity (Lash and Urry 1987; Giddens 1994).

Finally, it needs to be emphasised that the position of ethnic minorities is at the centre of these changes and is receiving increased attention in research on the links between social structure and health. As was seen in the earlier summary of research findings, a more complex picture emerges than a simple class analysis allows. To repeat the main point of the work by Andrews and Jewson mentioned earlier, data on mortality and ethnic origin shows 'a remarkable pattern of diversity and change ... that represents a challenge to many orthodox explanations for inequalities' (Andrews and Jewson 1993: 138).

Andrews and Jewson argue that 'effective explanations' for such health inequalities are likely to be found 'in the context of configurations of social relationships, including patterns of economic, political and power differentials' (Andrews and Jewson 1993: 142). Specifically, these authors point to the limits of applying the materialist approach from the Black Report in a simplistic form, if only because it has been found that some groups suffer high levels of deprivation and discrimination but have low levels of infant mortality. Without 'disaggregating measures of deprivation, the specific features that lead to health risks, and those which protect against such risks, will be missed' (Andrews and Jewson 1993: 145).

Future work, these authors suggest, will need to be designed 'with the distinctive economic, housing, household and other features of ethnic minority communities in mind, including the experience of racism' (Andrews and Jewson 1993: 147). In arguing for such an approach they reinforce the case put forward by Macintyre and Blaxter for a new direction in the field as a whole. While the evidence on inequalities in health may continue to be used to reinforce arguments for structural change and the reduction of wide disparities in wealth and income (Wilkinson 1996), a sociological perspective can also feed into the kind of policy development advocated by Vagero, where the needs of specific groups are examined for their more general 'public health significance' (Vagero 1995: 13). Equally important, perhaps, at least from the point of view of the argument of this book, is that such research will not only provide a more fine-grained view of health inequalities, but will also act as a window on critical features of social and cultural change.

Chapter 3

Doctors, patients and interaction in health care

INTRODUCTION

In the last twenty years, much of the academic and public debate about the Health Service (rather than 'health', as discussed in previous chapters) has focused on the nature of the 'doctor–patient relationship'. While this chapter also examines perspectives and evidence about this relationship, it does so at a time of significant change. Though it is clear that doctors are, in most cases, finally (and legally) responsible for treatment decisions and care in the health services, the doctor–patient relationship has tended to be regarded as an unchanging phenomenon. The idea that contact between doctors and patients should be described in terms of a 'relationship' is, in any event, a rather strange notion. We would not, for example, speak so easily of the dentist–patient relationship, or even of the nurse–patient relationship, though these terms are sometimes used. In fact, while the term 'doctor–patient relationship' has widespread currency, it probably emerged originally from medical circles, referring to the claim of doctors to have a special place in the health care system and thus a special 'relationship' with the patient. Put this way, the term seems more ideological than descriptive, rendering clinical judgement and medical claims over the patient benign, and conveying a 'medico-centric' image of trust and public acceptability. The use of the term in the medical sociology context may have always been more problematic than recognised, and this needs to be borne in mind in the subsequent discussion.

The term 'doctor–patient relationship' also has a particular historical ring in the UK context. The idea of *the* doctor–patient relationship has been particularly associated with the development of general practice, where traditionally individual doctors related to their patients over long periods of time, often for a lifetime. The pattern of the 'family doctor' who served all members of the household and who ran a single-handed practice (often administered by a spouse – invariably a wife) existed in the health services in Britain for several decades, and still exists in some local areas, especially rural ones. This form of 'relationship' with patients was associated with substantial 'out of hours' contact, and home visiting for births and deaths, as well as in times of illness.

For a while, such doctors continued to relate to 'their patients' even when clinical activities were being transferred to hospital settings; general practitioners would help in delivery wards (or GP maternity units) or visit patients admitted to hospital medical and surgical wards. In sociological terms, GPs were, in comparison with hospital doctors, more autonomous, and 'client oriented' rather than 'collegiate oriented' (Freidson 1989). In many respects they could be seen as running small businesses (Calnan and Gabe 1991). As we shall see, much of medical sociology research on the doctor–patient relationship developed in the context of emerging stresses in this pattern of UK general practice.

In recent years, partly as a result of these and other changes in the social relations of health care, sociologists have used the term 'doctor–patient relationship' less often. Medical sociologists now prefer to talk of 'lay–professional relationships' (Nettleton 1995) or in terms of 'the healing relationship: doctors, nurses and patients' (Radley 1994). These phrases signify a shift in attention towards a more pluralistic structure and outlook, and a relative displacement of the doctor from a central position in the analysis of the health care process. In turn, this approach to the role of doctors reflects the changing nature of professional power and authority more generally, which, though still significant, is now affected by a series of challenges from a variety of sources.

However, as indicated, the focus on doctor–patient relationships has been one of the key themes of medical sociology and is central to the present discussion. In order to evaluate the degree of change that has taken place in this area (including the extent of professional 'displacement'), a careful review of the development of research on the topic is therefore required. Initial interest among medical sociology researchers stemmed in large part from a series of pragmatic and policy concerns which developed in the UK, especially in the 1960s and 1970s, in general practice; hospital relationships also came under scrutiny. The research agenda was then concerned with such matters as 'compliance', the appropriate use of services, problems of communication and what appeared to be a developing sense of 'low morale' among doctors. Attempts to meet this with the development of teams in health centres were advocated (Jefferys and Sachs 1983). Allegations by doctors that patients were presenting too many 'trivial complaints' were frequent, though there was also a sense that patients were often too deferential in the consultation itself (Cartwright 1967; Cartwright and Anderson 1981).

Though some of these issues are less in evidence today than they once were, many remain important to the assessment of interactions in health care. As chapter 1 noted, protests by GPs about 'trivial' complaints can still be heard in the NHS. Indeed, most of the themes mentioned here, especially communication and the behaviour and expectations of patients, continue to feature strongly in health care evaluation. As was also discussed in chapter 1, British research on lay–professional encounters – especially in the hospital context – acted as a springboard for a wider appreciation of lay beliefs and knowledge about health and illness more generally.

In addition to these substantive issues, it should also be noted that interactions and relationships in health care have been of *theoretical* interest to sociologists, partly because they illustrate some of the major features of modern society. The position of doctors and patients exemplifies, in particular, the central place of professional authority and its acceptance or resistance by people who encounter it. The doctor–patient relationship is not only a major aspect of modern health care experience but also a critical lens through which the impact of scientific, technical and rational authority on everyday life can be observed. Though other relationships in health care are of growing importance, the doctor–patient relationship remains the one meeting point where, periodically for many but frequently for some, individuals encounter science and professional authority in their most developed and intimate form. In studying the doctor–patient relationship, medical sociology has therefore combined an interest in the political and pragmatic concerns of policy (e.g. standards in general practice) with concepts and ideas about power and authority.

Against this backdrop the present chapter proceeds by two main stages. The first section examines the three most important conceptual frameworks within which medical sociology research on the doctor–patient relationship has developed. This reiterates in a more focused form those perspectives that have informed most sociological work in the post-Second World War period, and which were outlined in the introduction to this book. A brief résumé may help at this point.

The first of these models is the *consensus model*, which is particularly associated with the work of Talcott Parsons. While there has been continuing interest in Parsons as a major theoretical influence in medical sociology (Gerhardt 1987, 1989) and as a theorist of 'modernity' (Holton and Turner 1986), Parsons' work has tended to be used, in practice, more as a critical foil than as a guide to empirical work. An analysis of Parsons' well-known views of the doctor–patient relationship remains important, however, as it addresses macro as well as micro issues concerning professional authority and social order.

The second model, developed in reaction to the notion of consensus in the doctor–patient relationship, is the *conflict model*. This is particularly associated with the work of Freidson and, as has already been shown, has considerably influenced British research. Rather than presuming consensus, this approach has set out to reveal the 'clash of perspectives' which is argued to be involved when doctors and patients meet. Where Parsons had seen difficulties in the doctor–patient relationship as being a function of poor role performance, Freidson saw conflict as a structural characteristic of a 'lay–professional' divide. Marxian and feminist versions of this critique are also identified.

The third model of the doctor–patient relationship to be discussed here is the *negotiation model* in which routine interactions have been seen to involve elements of both consensus and conflict. Drawing on the work of sociologists such as Goffman and Strauss, with their emphasis on the maintenance of order under conditions of change (see chapter 5), empirical studies within this model have stressed the active role patients play in the interactional setting. In this model the doctor–patient relationship is 'emergent'; the result of bargaining processes between the individuals concerned. While mindful, to varying degrees, of the structural differences between doctors and patients, this model suggests that the outcome of interaction is not wholly determined by them. Attention is also paid in such work to the importance of differences *between* doctors, in terms of their values and outlook on relationships with patients. In this model, the doctor–patient relationship is therefore treated as more of a contingent reality. In turn, this opens up the possibility of

regarding relationships in health care as being founded on participation or even a 'shared' basis.

In the second part of the chapter a series of challenges to the
doctor–patient relationship are discussed. While the models identified above remain relevant, enough has already been said to indicate
that the social context in which they are now being applied, and in
which they will be applied in the future, is changing rapidly. The
main features of these changes are discussed, as are their implications for future research on the doctor–patient relationship. Again,
a brief introductory note here may help the reader.

The first of these changes concerns illness (morbidity) patterns,
medical information and clinical care. As discussed elsewhere in this
book (especially chapter 4), the nature of 'patienthood' has altered
significantly in recent years. Not only has the population aged but
the increase in chronic illness has been accompanied by a tendency
for patients to be more knowledgeable about their condition than in
the past. Moreover, in the context of general practice, the patient
may now become an 'expert' in a situation where the doctor may
necessarily have only a general understanding of the disorder. The
possibilities and constraints of a more 'shared' approach to care in
such situations need to be considered.

Second, the chapter identifies changes in the nature of medical
authority and trust and the relative decline in patient deference.
These cultural developments have major implications for arguments
about medical dominance and the 'colonisation of the life world' of
the patient, on which conflict approaches particularly have been
based. The proliferation of 'discourses' on health and medicine can
be seen to displace the central authority of medicine in health
matters, aided and abetted by the growth of medical information
and media coverage. Challenges also emanate from new social
movements and campaigns around health issues, linked with such
developments as alternative medicine and counselling. These, in
turn, may be seen to result from the widespread adoption of what
might be called 'new age' or pluralistic values, especially among the
young, in which the place of professionals such as doctors (and thus
the doctor–patient relationship) may become particularly problematic.

In addition, this section of the chapter discusses the impact of
legal and ethical challenges to the doctor–patient relationship and
their implication for the autonomy of doctors. The spur to some of
these changes has come from a greater tendency to identify medical

negligence and malpractice and a greater public awareness of the limits or frontiers of medicine. The growth of complaints by patients which are dealt with within the health care system is also noteworthy. Consumerist and managerial challenges are also identified here, including those that now result from government policy; notable in the British context is the 'Patient's Charter' (DoH 1991), which has brought both government edict and managerial structures to bear on the doctor–patient relationship, laying down specific guidelines on a number of issues including such matters as out-patient waiting times. These changes, in particular, suggest that a 'contractual' and consumer-led doctor–patient relationship may now be emerging.

Third and finally, the chapter notes the extension of all of these developments through the increasing adoption of evaluative techniques which expose the doctor–patient relationship to increasing scrutiny. The new research issues which flow from this, and especially patient satisfaction research, are considered, and the question is posed of how far these should constitute the future medical sociology agenda in this area.

MODELS OF THE DOCTOR–PATIENT RELATIONSHIP

The consensus model

Talcott Parsons is often identified as the 'founding father' of medical sociology. Apart from the quaintness of this designation, it is not altogether accurate, as sociological studies of health and illness, especially mental illness in urban America, had been conducted throughout the decades before Parsons turned to the subject, and major studies of the subject were published in the 1950s (e.g. Hollingshead and Redlich 1958). What is true, however, is that in the same period Parsons developed for the first time a thoroughgoing *theoretical* account of health, illness and medicine. This formed part of an overall structural-functionalist theory of modern American society, which aimed to provide nothing less than a complete account of the 'functional prerequisites' of the social system and the 'needs dispositions' of people living in it. Central to this project, both theoretical and real, was the rapid rise in importance of the professions. For Parsons, following Max Weber, the professions represented a new form of 'legitimate authority', based on rational and scientific knowledge and on a 'collectivity orientation', in contradistinction to the more coercive form of 'business ethic' which had previously dominated American life (Parsons 1951: 535).

As a result, the professions featured prominently in Parsons' work, especially in discussions of education, social welfare and, of course, medicine. The doctor–patient relationship occupied a central position in this schema, allowing Parsons to examine a range of issues, from the dependency needs of the patient to the social control functions of the doctor. In this relationship, macro social structures could be seen to be embedded in the most focused of micro settings (the medical encounter) and in the most intimate of personal experiences (illness). In this sense, Parsons presented the first thoroughgoing account of illness and medicine as social rather than purely biological or 'natural' phenomena. For the purposes of this discussion the chapter will concentrate on the main lines of his argument, especially his well-known exposition of the doctor–patient relationship in chapter X of *The Social System* (Parsons 1951), together with his subsequent defence of his theory in a later essay (Parsons 1978).

One of the most important problems Parsons addressed is the question of how a relationship characterised by 'a-symmetry' could function as well as it appeared to do. Drawing on psychoanalytic thought, Parsons argued that the patient typically approaches the doctor in a state of distress and need (interestingly, 'need' as opposed to 'want' in the sense of the person in the market place, Parsons 1951: 440–441, 463), without either the knowledge or the ability to rectify the difficulties being experienced. In short, the patient is in a vulnerable and emotional state. The doctor, on the other hand, is placed in a powerful position over the patient, and may increase that power by intruding further into the patient's private life. For example, taboos surrounding access to the body may be broken and actions taken (e.g. investigations or surgery) that in other circumstances would either constitute assault or at least lead to considerable social friction, given the body's normal 'inviolability' (Parsons 1951: 451).

The answer to this, for Parsons, formed part of his general account of how inequality, or asymmetry in power and knowledge in modern social systems, could be reconciled with maintaining social order. The key lay in the ability of the system to fashion values and roles which could provide the necessary basis for a shared 'consensus' on what was proper conduct and what the goals of action were. In order to analyse these, Parsons advocated building a 'typology of social structure' (Parsons 1978: 21). In the case of the doctor–patient relationship, such structural characteristics were codified by Parsons in terms of the now well-known formulation of the 'sick role' for patient behaviour and the 'physician role', within a 'collegial form of association', for acting appropriately as a doctor. It is important, as Gerhardt has pointed out, in seeking to understand the significance of the sick role in particular, not to divorce these ideas from the wider framework within which Parsons fashioned them (Gerhardt 1979).

As far as the conduct component of the equation is concerned, doctors and patients need to orientate themselves towards each other in a trustful manner. Though Parsons frequently contrasted the doctor–patient relationship with that obtaining in business circles, he also referred to the doctor–patient relationship as a 'fiduciary' one (Parsons 1978: 24), borrowing the term from the world of banking and finance: here, trust has to be based on abstract codes of conduct in circumstances where no exchange of goods is actually taking place. In order to establish such trust with patients, doctors must, according to Parsons, behave towards patients in an 'affectively neutral' manner. In other words, they must resist emotional involvement, favouritism and the negative aspects of 'transference' which may occur in the clinical encounter. Moreover, as noted, the doctor should also display a 'collectivity orientation' in which the good of the patient is seen to be paramount, and where pecuniary interests are excluded from the immediate confines of the encounter.

As far as patients are concerned, they must, according to Parsons, adopt and display certain behaviours in being, or acting, 'sick'. Most notable are the needs to show that illness is regarded as undesirable and that the patient will co-operate willingly with the doctor. These show the necessary disposition by patients in conducting themselves with doctors, such as to convince the latter that the necessary norms and rules of the encounter are understood and that trust is established. From this viewpoint it is possible to see why so much attention has been given by doctors to compliance and the appropriate amount of deference by patients: that is, to the performance of patients in following 'doctors' orders' (specifically, completing treatment programmes in order to get well) when the patient is no longer under the direct surveillance of the doctor (Parsons 1951: 437).

In return for displaying these positive modes of conduct, the patient, too, is then accorded certain rights. These are temporary release from social obligations and a release from responsibility for falling ill. Parsons saw that illness presents a particular form of 'deviance': although the person may not be thought of as responsible for their action, some degree of 'motivation' towards illness could be present, if not in terms of initial occurrence (though this may be the case in differential exposure to risk, Parsons 1951: 430) then in terms of its maintenance. In this sense being sick is a 'negatively achieved role' resulting from the failure to keep well (Parsons 1951: 438). Release from responsibility counters the possible charge that others may make to claims by the sick person for special dispensation, especially that of malingering.

The goals of the doctor–patient relationship flow from this, and are themselves underpinned by normative structures. In essence, the goal of the doctor–patient relationship is to try to ensure that the state of 'sickness' is temporary and to reintegrate the person back into their normal social roles as soon as possible. For this reason patients are required not only to want to get well but also to recognise illness as an undesirable state. This latter point may seem obvious from a medical or common-sense viewpoint. But such is the nature of illness and the complex psychological and social dispositions it brings forth that, Parsons argues, the therapeutic encounter will only be 'functional' or 'consensual' if the perception of regaining positive health (and thus the need for medical intervention) is clearly understood. In this way treating illness is part of the normative structure and socialisation process of the individual, and is central to the 'patterned roles' of the social system (Parsons 1951: 433–434).

It has been argued that these views of the doctor–patient relationship have been particularly important to an understanding of medicine's role as a form of social control in modern society (Gerhardt 1989: 49–50). As has been shown, the doctor–patient relationship and therapy are seen by Parsons to involve powerful forms of reward and sanction. These were key aspects of social learning processes which Parsons thought were central to social life (ibid.). Nevertheless, Parsons' approach to this and other issues has been the focus of sustained sociological criticism ever since publication. Indeed, much of the development of medical sociology's interest in the doctor–patient relationship can be seen as a series of responses and challenges to Parsons' arguments.

At this point, one criticism in particular should be noted, which is central to understanding Parsons' attachment to the consensus model of the doctor–patient relationship. This is the tendency of his approach to portray sickness as a temporary phenomenon. It is this feature on which much of Parsons' theorising depends. If sickness is temporary, doctors and patients can work together towards the common goal of 'returning the patient to normal', allowing the various rights and obligations to come into play in the expectation that they will be limited in application. For example, the patient may only be willing, or happy, to be released from obligations (e.g. paid work) if these obligations are held in temporary suspension, pending return. Similarly, doctors may only be allowed to break the taboo of access to the body if it is also circumscribed and temporary. The more these temporary features are eroded the more difficult the relationship would appear to become. Social order, here, is conceived as a set of checks and balances, based on a circumscribed and 'functionally specific' use of authority.

As Gallagher (1976), among others, has argued, however, chronic illness now dominates the worlds of both doctors and patients. Gallagher asks how it is possible, in these circumstances, to reconcile Parsons' picture of temporary deviance and the 'safety valve' of the sick role with the preponderance of chronic illness. He states:

> In chronic illness exemption from normal social role obligations cannot be justified by the prospect of a return to productive function and social participation. Neither can the obligation to seek treatment or to cooperate with treatment orders be so justified.

(Gallagher 1976: 209)

This is often quoted as a telling criticism of the sick role theory, especially as it also points to the empirical realities of illness in contrast to Parsons' somewhat abstract theorising. It is especially important when ageing is taken into account; the retired elderly do not have the same 'role set' as younger people. However, Parsons provides a straightforward reply in his later essay. In the case of chronic illness (and even terminal illness) he argues that 'the goal of complete recovery becomes impractical' (Parsons 1978: 18), and agrees that the full repertoire of the sick role may not be applicable in such circumstances. This admission goes at least part way to meeting Gallagher's point about the limited scope of the sick role concept.

But Parsons maintains that in many instances (and here he uses the example of diabetes, from which he suffered himself) 'deterioration can be held in check by the proper medically prescribed measures based on sound diagnostic knowledge' (Parsons 1978: 19). On the patient's side 'adhering to a proper regimen and deferring to a proper medical authority' helps maintain key elements of the sick role. Though previous activities may not be fully recovered, the patient is still obliged to maintain normal physical functioning 'and as many activities of life' as possible (ibid.). In this way Parsons argued that his approach to the doctor–patient relationship could be applied to chronic illness situations without a great deal of difficulty. The consensus model could thus still be seen to be relevant, even in circumstances which were different from those (i.e. acute illness) on which it was based. Social order could be maintained through longer-term, though still circumscribed, use of doctors' authority. Attempts to outline an 'impairment role', for example (Gordon 1966), had already extended Parsons' views in a more empirical direction in an attempt to take account of these factors. However, if this extension is at least partly granted, a functionalist view of the doctor–patient relationship retains other more fundamental difficulties, and it is these that the conflict and negotiation models have sought to address.

The conflict model

Parsons himself was aware that the doctor–patient relationship, like many others in modern life, was problematic. For example, though modern medical practice was based on scientific knowledge, Parsons saw that this was often incomplete or uncertain. Moreover, poor knowledge on the part of doctors and patients could lead to poor 'role performance' in which either party might not play their role in a competent manner. Even so, such difficulties, for Parsons, did not detract from his basic view that doctor–patient relationships were based on trust and consensus.

As has been seen, this was part of a theoretical elaboration of the role of professional authority in modern (American) society. As chapter 1 has discussed, during the 1960s and 1970s other, more critical views of this authority, and thus of the doctor–patient relationship, began to emerge. Foremost in the assault on Parsons, at least from a medical sociology viewpoint, was Eliot Freidson. His book *Profession of Medicine* (1970a), which drew on the 'social

construction of reality' of Berger and Luckmann (1967) combined
with elements of labelling and conflict theory, set out to challenge
the functionalist view of professional activity handed down by
Parsons. Where Parsons saw legitimate authority and trust,
Freidson saw 'medical dominance' and suppressed conflict. And
while Parsons saw the social control functions of medicine and the
doctor–patient relationship as having positive outcomes, Freidson,
in contrast, saw them as far from therapeutic.

The main problem for Freidson was that as patients and doctors
inhabited different social and cultural worlds and were concerned
with different realities – patients with illness and doctors with
disease – conflict was likely to be a structural feature, not simply a
function of poor role performance. Arguing against Parsons, and
specifically against the emphasis on a functional 'mutual participation' approach in models of the doctor–patient relationship such as
those of Szasz and Hollander (1956), Freidson states:

> Given the two viewpoints of the two worlds, lay and profes-
> sional, in interaction, they can never be wholly synonymous. And
> they are always, if only latently, in conflict. Indeed I wish to
> suggest that the most faithful perspective on interaction in treat-
> ment is one reflecting such conflict in standpoint, not on
> assuming an identity of purpose to be discovered by better
> education or a disposition to cooperate sometimes hidden by
> misunderstanding or by failure to cooperate.
>
> (Freidson 1970a: 321–322)

Such an approach to doctor–patient interaction opened up for
many medical sociologists a new and more challenging chapter for
research. As has been noted, the doctor–patient relationship was
already being studied empirically, particularly in the context of
general practice. Studies based on survey work, such as that of
Cartwright and O'Brien (1976), showed that social class variations
in consulting patterns bore out the contention that no simple 'identity of purpose' could be observed. At the least, the manner of
achieving it varied considerably, depending on key social factors.
Clear differences in the amount of time doctors spent with working-
class and middle-class patients, for example, and the more passive
role of the former, suggested that the doctor–patient relationship
was structured in socially significant ways. Stimson's (1976) survey
of general practitioners' views found that, far from exhibiting a
'collectivity orientation' and 'affective neutrality', doctors found

little difficulty reporting which kinds of patients they liked and did not like. Women, especially those with children, and patients with emotional and psychological illnesses were reported as particularly 'troublesome'. Far from social life being based on shared values and legitimate authority, this kind of work suggested that, at best, it rested on an uneasy mixture of hidden conflict and differences in outlook.

Other research began to draw more explicitly on Freidson's views of conflict in examining relationships in general practice. Bloor and Horobin (1975), for example, took Freidson as their point of departure in challenging head-on Parsons' 'reciprocal' view of the doctor–patient relationship. With growing evidence showing not only social variations in consulting behaviour but also dissatisfaction among doctors about their patients' behaviour, including such issues as demanding too many night calls, a conflict approach appeared to have much to commend it (Bloor and Horobin 1975: 276).

Using Schutz's notion of 'typification' and its role in social life as well as Freidson's views of conflict, Bloor and Horobin went on to argue that doctors, especially GPs, operated with a contradictory view of patient behaviour. On the one hand, the typical patient is supposed to be a 'well informed citizen' who knows when it is appropriate to consult the doctor. On the other hand, the same patient should 'defer to the opinion of the doctor' once in the consultation room (Bloor and Horobin 1975: 277). Hence the role prescription for the patient, they argued, turns out to be contradictory, constituting a 'double bind' in which the 'sick person is first encouraged to participate in and then excluded from the therapeutic relationship' (ibid.).

For these authors, frustration and conflict in the doctor–patient relationship stem from two sources. The first of these is that doctors expect patients to 'assess their disorder' before coming to see the doctor, without realising that this may conflict with their own assessment in the consultation (Bloor and Horobin 1975: 279). Second, in expecting patients to defer to their opinion in the consultation, doctors convey the idea that patients' ideas are of little value. This may actually discourage them from properly assessing their condition prior to consultation (ibid.). While the conflict produced by these contradictory expectations may not always be overt, frustration may only be held in check by the precarious mechanisms of 'impression management' and the deference of the patient. By recognising the power imbalance in the situation, the patient 'may decide to steer clear of potential conflict on the grounds that such conflicts are distressing and undesirable' (Bloor and Horobin 1975: 280). This situation is clearly a far cry from Parsons' consensual views, and demands, according to Bloor and Horobin, that the underlying structural reasons for conflict need to be identified rather than ways of reducing it as 'an end in itself' (Bloor and Horobin 1975: 281).

While general practice was a particularly important site for the debate about conflict and consensus in the doctor–patient relationship in Britain, it should be noted that studies have not been confined to this arena. Mention has already been made of the fact that work on patient views of illness in Britain began with research which focused on interaction within the hospital setting (see chapter 1). In the US, work on the doctor–patient relationship has been particularly concerned, as Freidson was, with hospital dynamics.

Waitzkin (1979), for example, sought to draw links between the 'micro' world of doctor–patient interaction and the wider structures of a capitalist society. Though Parsons also sought to draw such links, as has been shown, his view of American capitalism was essentially positive. In contrast, and in an argument drawing upon Marxian ideas, Waitzkin interpreted routine hospital medical encounters as a means of reinforcing dominant ideologies rather than helping to reinforce shared values. The medical encounter, he held, de-politicises the effects of capitalist social relations, especially of work, in producing illness and rendering the patient inactive and 'mute' in challenging oppressive conditions (Waitzkin 1979, 1984; see also Mishler 1984 for a similar line of argument).

In a series of responses to Waitzkin's views a number of British medical sociologists sought to distance themselves from this approach to conflict theory. Rayner and Stimson, for example, argued that Waitzkin's approach was far too mechanistic to stand up to serious scrutiny. In particular, there was no attempt in his analysis, they argued, to explore whether the encounters he described were specific to the political context of American capitalism and medicine at that time in comparison with European settings (Rayner and Stimson 1979: 611). Strong made a similar point by asking whether the interactions observed by Waitzkin were common to all medical encounters, and whether it was legitimate to 'read off' macro implications from micro encounters (Strong 1979c: 613). The exchange between Waitzkin and his critics is of note, if only because it illustrates that, despite the influence of the conflict perspective, this has often stopped short, in British medical sociology, of embracing Marxist versions.

At the same time, however, feminist writings were arguing for a clear critical perspective, analysing 'male domination' in the medical encounter, especially in the context of obstetric and maternity care. Work was also conducted on the experience of women in the context of general practice. For example, in a frequently cited paper, Barrett and Roberts (1978) argued that doctors treated women in stereotypical ways, and, like Waitzkin, argued that exchanges between individual doctors and patients revealed the ways in which dominant assumptions about social relations – in this case, traditional women's roles – were reproduced in the doctor–patient relationship. Deference among the female patients being studied was taken as a sign of (male) medical dominance rather than genuine satisfaction with care. This was followed up in a further publication by Roberts (1985) in which she argued, again, that general practitioner encounters with their female patients were characterised by a tendency to reinforce assumptions about their social roles, compromising an independent view of their clinical needs.

In a series of influential papers and books, Oakley also argued against the promulgation of male control over the care of women, again especially in childbirth (Oakley 1980, 1984). In *Women Confined* (1980) Oakley argued that the medicalisation of childbirth excluded alternative practices that would give women more control over the process, regarding them as 'deviant and esoteric' (Oakley 1980: 216). In the medical encounter, such medicalisation often meant that 'the patient's attitude to pregnancy is ignored by the examining doctor, who instead focuses his and the patient's attention narrowly on its medical management' (Oakley 1980: 30). Her study of 66 women going through hospital delivery showed various aspects of care, including doctor–patient interaction in a critical light. However, the study also found that only a minority of women expressed opinions about adopting an alternative approach. Most women were satisfied with the management of their birth (Oakley 1980: 123). Oakley attempted to reconcile this with her more critical perspective in the following way:

At the moment, it is not possible to produce research findings that show that the majority of women are dissatisfied with medical styles of childbirth management – in the sense of wanting a radically different alternative to medicalized birth. But, on the other hand, many studies, including this one, do demonstrate a great deal of discontent.

(Oakley 1980: 216)

Although, as we shall see below, feminist critiques of the doctor–patient relationship, as taken up by the women's movement, have continued to constitute a major challenge to the consensus perspective, much medical sociology has remained cautious of a 'strong' conflict programme, partly because of observed levels of 'expressed satisfaction' with care. As Stimson and Strong made clear, however, one of the theoretical reasons for such caution is also the attachment of British medical sociologists to an interpretive view of social interaction, which does not lend itself to broad structural generalisations and is wary of overstating the 'medicalisation' thesis. As indicated, both Marxist and feminist critiques found difficulties in arguing (in somewhat different ways) that conflict was at the root of doctor–patient relationships, when patients were often observed valuing the care they had received.

The negotiation model

From the viewpoint of interpretive medical sociology, separating a negotiation model from a conflict model of doctor–patient relationships is difficult. In reality, the idea of negotiation presumes a degree of conflict and vice versa. Indeed, Freidson argued for the adoption of a negotiation model based on the idea of 'offers and responses' being made in the clinical setting, that had earlier been put forward by the psychoanalyst Michael Balint (Freidson 1970a: 322). Negotiation implies both the presence of conflict and the willingness to work towards an agreement, if not in establishing a consensus.

In effect, a negotiation model plays down 'structural constraints' in order to emphasise the more contingent nature of social interaction. Both consensus and conflict may be present, but neither are likely to prevail except under specific circumstances. For example, the doctor–patient relationship may change over time, as interactions occur at different stages of an illness trajectory. The relationship may also be affected by the contingencies of the type of illness and the organisation of the health care setting, as well as by social factors such as age, class, gender, ethnicity and so on. The negotiation model suggests that the researcher should bring to the fore the ways relationships are configured, maintained and changed without either consensus or conflict being a predictable outcome.

One of the clearest examples of a negotiation approach to the doctor–patient relationship is that of Stimson and Webb's (1975) study *Going to See the Doctor*. Because of the range of issues raised in this study and their lasting relevance to the negotiation approach, the following discussion presents their findings in some detail.

Observations and recorded consultations and interviews with 96 patients were carried out in two South Wales general practices. The authors were able to build up a detailed picture of the 'emergent' nature of doctor–patient relationships, focusing on the processes before encounters, those during the consultations and reactions after the event.

Before the consultation, Stimson and Webb showed how the patient (or 'proto patient', to use Bloor and Horobin's term) deals with the uncertainty of whether to consult and what the appropriate use of the service is. Advice from others within the person's 'social network' and expectations of what the doctor may do as a result of consulting influence this decision-making. Expectations may involve consideration of whether doctors will provide emotional support or additional resources, including access to specialist treatment (Stimson and Webb 1975: 22). In fact, the authors commented, patient expectations are difficult to unravel, partly because though the patient may be weighing up the expected benefits and costs of consulting, these may not be easy to predict.

Stimson and Webb also discussed the degree and nature of the preparation patients make before consulting. This may involve the *rehearsal* of what is to be said, as a way of reducing the power imbalance between doctor and patient in the consultation. It may also involve such matters as picking up cues about the situation in the waiting-room, including how late the session is running and even what mood the doctor is in (Stimson and Webb 1975: 35).

In the 'face-to-face' interaction Stimson and Webb argued that both doctors and patients employ strategies and negotiation tactics. In this sense, patients are not merely passive partners in the process. Of course, this does not mean that the outcome can easily be determined by the patient, if at all, but it does suggest that it is more 'emergent' and negotiable than either the consensus or conflict models allow. In the interactions observed, patients were seen deliberately to select what they wanted to say, just as doctors did, and both interrupted the speech of the other (Stimson and Webb 1975: 43). Patients were also seen to select the mode of presentation of information, especially in emphasising the serious-ness of a problem, or by trying to ensure that it was dealt with before other matters were discussed.

According to Stimson and Webb, patients may also try to influ-ence the consultation process by expressing dissatisfaction with prior decisions, though this is rarely in terms of outright criticism of the doctor (as Bloor and Horobin argued). In part, this is because patients know that doctors hold the 'trump card' of providing access to further treatment or resources. Time pressures also work in favour of the doctor, in that patients are aware or accept the idea of not taking up the doctor's time (Stimson and Webb 1975: 59). However, even the termination of the consultation is not wholly within the control of the doctor. Though the 'time honoured tech-niques' of moving from the chair and rising to one's feet were frequently employed by the doctors, patients were also seen to control the end of the interaction, especially by reducing or increasing their responses to the doctor's questions or statements.

One of the main contributions of this study was to emphasise the importance, in the doctor–patient relationship, of events following the consultation. While earlier research had stressed deference and passivity of patients, especially during the consultation, Stimson and Webb pointed to the 'countervailing power' patients could muster outside. Patients were observed making judgements about the results of the consultation some time after its completion, some-times by recounting 'atrocity stories'. This often allowed them to return to their own frame of reference and social network. Other people within such networks were shown to play an important role in judging the outcomes. Stimson and Webb state that 'Information acquired even several weeks or months later may throw light on the consultation and lead to further interpretation of what went on' (Stimson and Webb 1975: 72).

In group discussions with patients, Stimson and Webb found a variety of reactions to the consultations. Some people were 'agree-ably surprised' at the result, while others felt 'thwarted' by the consultation, especially when being sent away with an unwanted prescription. On many occasions, however, reappraisal of the consultation was not a straightforward matter. People began to formulate their expectations only after the event. Interestingly, in the light of today's research agenda, this led Stimson and Webb to ask how 'patient satisfaction' might be operationalised in research. For them the problem lay in appreciating the 'fluctuating nature of people's feelings about their encounters with doctors' rather than in adopting more structured questionnaire techniques (Stimson and Webb 1975: 77). Patients might feel satisfied with some aspects of doctors' actions but not others, and this, they argued, cuts across classifying patients' responses in terms of 'levels of satisfaction' (Stimson and Webb 1975: 78).

Patient satisfaction research will be returned to below. For the moment, however, it needs to be emphasised that Stimson and Webb's study showed that there is no simple relationship between doctors' actions, patient expectations and the outcomes of the consultation, in terms of either compliance or satisfaction. The negotiation model suggests, however, that in general practice in particular, although patients may not be able to determine the outcome of the consultation in any simple way, they may have considerable ability to control events (and thus redress the power imbalance) after the event.

As was argued in chapter 1, part of the attraction of an interactionist model of behaviour for sociologists has been its emphasis, in contrast to both functionalist and conflict perspectives, of the active nature of the 'social actor'. Subsequent research, in a variety of health care settings, has documented the ways in which the patient can be seen as active, albeit in a 'negative' way. For example, Bloor and McIntosh (1990) have documented how avoidance and concealment techniques may be employed by patients in resisting surveillance exercised by health care professionals. The empirical data for their discussion are taken from earlier studies of social processes in 'therapeutic communities' and in health visiting. In examining concealment strategies by patients in the former setting, they show how 'deviant conformity' can allow patients to appear to be following orders while secretly subverting them (Bloor and McIntosh 1990: 177). In the latter setting, they show how avoidance can be employed by mothers using simple devices such as not attending clinics or not answering the door when the health visitor calls on them at home (Bloor and McIntosh 1990: 175).

Silverman (1987), in a study of 'going private', also showed how different settings could influence patient experiences and actions. In comparing medical encounters in NHS and private practices, he showed that patients in the latter settings could more positively initiate exchanges with the doctor and obtain a more 'personalised service'. This was often held back in the NHS setting by a hierarchical and bureaucratic ethos. However, a more active stance by the patient in the private setting was weighed against a lack of back-up services, such as radiology and pathology (Silverman 1987: 131).

Such studies suggested that the doctor–patient or professional–client relationship could be less hierarchical and more co-operative in character if only patients' views (and their active involvement in treatment) were taken more seriously. Again, such a perspective offers a challenge to both consensual and conflict models, both of which tend to view the patient as passive. However, few studies have systematically examined whether doctors are prepared to move in this direction or whether a more explicit negotiated approach is in fact feasible. An exception, again in the general practice context, is that carried out by Tuckett and his colleagues (Tuckett et al. 1985). The basic aim of this study was to examine whether a more equal sharing of ideas was a realistic prospect for the doctor–patient relationship. The study concentrated on the actions of 16 doctors, 8 of whom had expressed an interest in communication problems and 8 of whom acted as a comparison group. Thirteen hundred consultations were recorded, 405 being analysed in depth, with 328 of the patients involved being subsequently interviewed after the consultation (Tuckett et al. 1985: 27, 31). The results of this extensive research project are worth considering at this point.

At first sight the results did not seem to be encouraging, from the point of view of the authors of the book. Doctors' behaviour in the consultation did not appear to involve active negotiation with patients, and doctors rarely discussed psychological or social dimensions of patients' problems, or ask about or respond to patients' ideas. Moreover, variations in time spent with patients and in styles of communication were difficult to explain on medical grounds alone (Tuckett et al. 1985: 76).

At the same time, the study also showed that patients were far from passive in the consultation. At least half of the consultations examined by the researchers showed clear evidence of attempts by patients to influence the sharing of information, though 'formulating ideas in the heat of the moment' proved to be difficult against a background of expectations of deference on part of both doctors and patients (Tuckett et al. 1985: 111–112). Difficulties in communication were largely the result of an 'absence of mutual exchange' rather than the presence of conflict (Tuckett *et al.* 1985: 166).

In contrast to Stimson and Webb, therefore, Tuckett *et al.* found, ten years on, a less dynamic picture in general practice. Most of the exchanges they recorded tended towards what they called a 'stereotypical' form, in which the doctor provided a considerable level of explanation but failed to listen to what patients had to say or to take much interest in exploring patients' views. While the interaction between doctor and patient was not characterised by either consensus or conflict, the resulting 'negotiation' was of a rather mundane character compared with the more 'lively' picture painted by Stimson and Webb. This may be partly the result of differences in methodology. While Stimson and Webb provided an interpretive exploration of patients' views, Tuckett *et al.*'s more quantitative approach may have had the effect of underplaying what patients actually thought. However, Tuckett *et al.*'s study offers a necessary corrective to overstating the active involvement of patients. While patients may express a range of views about doctors, both before and after the consultation, Tuckett *et al.* show that the actual negotiation is often marked by a relatively low level of mutual involvement.

The conclusion drawn from this study, that patients are not treated as 'experts' in their own health care (Tuckett *et al.* 1985: 211), underlines the point that a systematic appreciation of patients' 'ideas, explanations and opinions' (ibid.) will not automatically characterise doctor–patient interactions just because they are seen as being part of a negotiation process. It is only when such negotiations are set within a framework that *explicitly* aims to achieve a more 'shared care' approach, and in which patients' actions are recognised as positive, that this may be achieved. The study proposes changes in professional commitment and education in order to challenge the persistent hierarchical structures within medicine. The authors also suggest that greater patient awareness is necessary if this is to be achieved. Recent research on relationships in hospital settings has also shown slow progress in achieving a shared approach, highlighting poor and unsympathetic communication by doctors (Audit Commission 1993). Condition-specific work, for example on stroke, has underlined the additional point that patients' relatives, as well as patients, may be excluded from adequate communication with doctors (Pound *et al.* 1995). As the chapter now goes on to discuss, however, a number of changes are under way which may give impetus to the emergence of a more 'shared' if still ambiguous doctor–patient relationship.

CHALLENGES TO THE DOCTOR–PATIENT RELATIONSHIP

Important though the models discussed above have been in highlighting key features of the doctor–patient relationship, they have one characteristic in common which limits their development. This is that they do not address clearly the issue of social change. Each of the models reviewed above discusses the doctor–patient relationship within the context of modern medical practice, but makes little reference to the changing environment in which this has taken place. Though the negotiation model suggests that patients may play a more active role, even this approach makes little or no reference to the changing cultural and policy context in which doctors and patients operate. Doubtless, part of the explanation for this may lie in the fact that during the period when most sociological research on the doctor–patient relationship was undertaken, the agenda was dominated by attempts to *propose* change rather than to report on it. Nevertheless, the doctor–patient relationship has been surprisingly decontextualised in much of the literature.

The situation today can be seen as substantially different from that which prevailed during the 1970s and most of the 1980s. Towards the end of the 1980s, it was possible to observe professional–patient relationships operating within an emerging *contractual model*, in which both doctors and patients might expect different patterns of behaviour and outlook from each other. In this model a more explicit recognition of what both parties can offer would be made. The doctor would provide clear information about treatment options and about the risks and benefits involved. The patient, in turn, would offer to assess the information, be willing to ask pertinent questions and accept a greater level of responsibility in accepting or refusing treatment.

At the beginning of this chapter three sources of change were identified which have particular implications for the doctor–patient relationship, and which might foster such a model. To remind the reader, these are: changes in illness patterns, especially the growing importance of chronic illness; the decline of both medical authority (resulting from the diffusion of medical information) and the influence of social movements, as well as the growth of legal, managerial and consumerist challenges to medicine; and, finally, the rapid increase in the evaluation of health care, linked to notions of accountability.

There is only space to sketch out these wide-ranging develop-ments in outline. Taken together, however, they can be seen as a major challenge to existing patterns of the doctor–patient relation-ship. They also signal transferral of power towards other professional groups, including nurses, lawyers and especially managers. How far these processes will benefit patients is a moot point. But at the least they suggest the need for a change in the medical sociology research agenda. Each of them is now discussed in turn.

Changes in illness patterns

As has been noted earlier in the discussion on Parsons' views and as the next chapter discusses in more detail, chronic illness now domi-nates the illness profile of late modern societies. Associated in part with an ageing population structure, this pattern of illness has several important implications for the doctor–patient relationship. The most important of these, as Gerhardt (1989) makes clear, is the shift from expectations of cure and patient compliance with treat-ment to an emphasis on the *management* of health disorders by doctors and patients alike. The long-term management of illness, and especially chronic illness, increasingly requires the sharing of ideas and the 'mutual expertise' of both doctors and patients.

In a study of the hospital management of chronic back pain, Fitzpatrick *et al.* (1987), for example, have demonstrated that patients may have a variety of different expectations of doctors and treatment and express different levels of satisfaction with care. In the study group in question, older patients, and those for whom contact with the doctor was for the first time, had rela-tively low expectations of 'cure', and wanted the doctor to provide reassurance and help, especially with managing pain and disability in everyday life. Middle-class patients, and those with more experience and knowledge of the treatment of back pain, were likely to be more critical of both the technical and interper-sonal aspects of care. Just under a third of the patients expressed dissatisfaction with discussions of their worries about the future of their condition (Fitzpatrick *et al.* 1987: 163). Many patients had a clear view of the possibilities and limits of the medical management of back pain and wished their views to be taken seriously.

Other studies of specific chronic disorders have underlined the growing expertise of patients in the daily management of the conditions. Schneider and Conrad's study of epilepsy (1983), Kelleher's study of diabetes (1988), I. Robinson's study of multiple sclerosis (1988) and Kelly's study of colitis (1992) all paint a similar picture in this regard. These studies report that though uncertainty may characterise patients' initial experience, and therefore their approach to doctors, this frequently gives way to a more confident stance once everyday management routines are established and as they learn more about the disorder and treatment options. Moreover, the active involvement of patients is partly dictated by the form of treatment. Increasingly, modern medical treatments *require* the active co-operation of patients for their success.

Kelly (1992), for example, shows how a 'contractual' relationship with the doctor develops as patients approach the possibility of surgery for colitis. Initially, patients may use a variety of techniques of avoidance and resistance to the idea of surgery. With time and through exchanges with surgeons, however, agreement is reached on how to proceed (Kelly 1992: 55–57). I. Robinson (1988) also shows that multiple sclerosis patients undertake considerable 'experimentation' with drug regimens before a strategy is found which is acceptable to themselves and their doctors. While these studies are largely based on interactions in the hospital sector, where negotiations about treatment may be more focused, the effect on future relationships with general practitioners should not be overlooked.

With the rapid increase in information available to patients, covering specific disorders as well as general health promotion, and with the growing importance of self-help groups, the processes of patient negotiation and active management of illness are likely to increase. Though research may still reveal the persistence of deference among patients in routine encounters, this may disguise a far more active outlook among specific groups of chronically ill or disabled patients. As patients' confidence and experience in managing long-term disorders rises, it can be expected that this will move the doctor–patient relationship in a less medically dominated direction. The potential for both conflict and co-operation in such circumstances is considerable. Linked to this are equally important changes in the position of the doctor as a central source of information and authority concerning illness and its treatment.

Medical authority in late modern cultures

As has been shown, the ideas of a reciprocal, conflictual or negotiated basis to the doctor–patient relationship all rely on an assumption of unequal access to medical knowledge and information. Whether a Parsonian or Freidsonian framework is adopted, each assumes that doctors have knowledge and power about disease and that patients are disadvantaged through lack of such knowledge. The differences in the various models of the doctor–patient relationship lie in their evaluation of this disparity; for Parsons it is essentially therapeutic, for Freidson, negative and potentially damaging. As noted, attempts by writers such as Tuckett *et al.* (1985) to portray the patient as an 'expert' seem confounded by the lack of clear empirical support showing either doctors or patients willing to recognise this routinely.

Yet a nascent contractual model can be detected, and not simply in the context of managing chronic health disorders. Most importantly, such a model is emerging from the long-term trend in the reduction of the power of professionals, related to the erosion of hierarchical relationships in late modern cultures more generally. It is possible to identify at least some of the factors which help explain the processes at work, especially in relation to the doctor–patient relationship.

As has been argued throughout this book, medical sociology writings have frequently argued (and sometimes overstated) that 'medical dominance' and 'medicalisation' have increasingly characterised modern society. The term 'medicalisation', especially popular in the American literature, refers to the process by which 'nonmedical problems become defined and treated as medical problems' (Conrad 1992: 209). Examples such as the menopause and dyslexia seem to testify to the process, first outlined by Irving Zola, in which 'more and more of life has come under medical dominance, influence and supervision' (Conrad 1992: 210; Zola 1972).

Yet today a number of paradoxes emerge when discussing this process. First, as Conrad himself notes, 'demedicalisation' is also occurring, where issues that were once part of medicine's remit no longer are (for example, the 'treatment' of homosexuality as a disease). Second, a number of studies have also shown in recent years that *patients* may demand a medical label when doctors are reluctant to do so. Disorders such as repetitive strain injury (RSI), chronic fatigue syndrome (CFS) and 'Gulf War' syndrome are cases in point. Here, the pressure on doctors to label ill-defined symptoms as diseases may significantly alter the doctor–patient relationship and erode the distinction between health and illness. Paradoxically, doctors may seek to resist the demand for a medical label if they cannot separate the disorder from the patient's account, and patients may feel frustrated if their accounts appear not to be taken seriously (Davey 1996). This process is frequently linked, on the patient's side, to the need for medical legitimation of claims to benefits, for example compensation or social security payments in RSI (Arksey 1994).

Equally significant, in the present context, is the fact that as medical knowledge expands and becomes widely disseminated its central place in managing health disorders actually declines, as doctors find it increasingly difficult to maintain their privileged control over it. As Giddens (1991) has pointed out in a more general sociological discussion of late modern cultures, expanding expertise may lead not only to the 'de-skilling' of lay people and the 'sequestration' of experience from everyday life (one facet of which is medicalisation) but also to a 're-skilling' in which people become active and 'empowered' (Giddens 1991: 138). So while medical expertise may reduce lay people's confidence in the face of illness, new forms of information and action (e.g. participating in self-help groups) may help them to restore a sense of control.

In fact, Giddens goes on to use a fictional medical scenario to illustrate the point. Interestingly, he asks his readers to consider the situation of a woman suffering from back pain. Giddens argues that she might, in Britain at least, first consult her GP, who in turn might refer her to a specialist. This might not be entirely satisfactory for the woman, particularly if the consultation does not lead to the offer of effective help. As has been seen above, this may well be true for a number of such patients. In any event, Giddens argues, treatment options need to be weighed up, especially if they involve the suggestion of surgery. The woman in question might, in doing this, also investigate alternative modes of treatment, including 'massage, acupuncture, exercise therapy, reflexology . . . the Alexander method, drug therapies, diet therapies, hands on healing – and no doubt other therapeutic modes also' (Giddens 1991: 140). At this point the woman might read into some of the medical literature on back pain. At the end of this process, 'a reasonably informed choice can in fact be made', even if it is to conclude that nothing much can be done to help (Giddens 1991: 141). The important point for Giddens, though, is that such decision-making is typically done today, 'with no overarching authority to whom she may turn – a characteristic dilemma in conditions of high modernity' (ibid.).

While medical sociologists might wish to test such suggestions against empirical evidence, the point being made is an important one. Both doctors and patients, in contemporary societies, must make decisions against a backcloth of a massive information explosion and pluralistic structures. Under such circumstances the notion of *the* doctor–patient relationship increasingly reflects the more settled period in the social relations of health care (and in society more generally) that characterised the 1950s and 1960s. Today, this relationship is frequently only one of a number that people may form in tackling health and illness issues, forming part of a more 'reflexive' and pluralistic social structure.

Part of the process being discussed here is, of course, affected by the enormous influence of the mass media. As Karpf (1988) has shown, throughout the 1940s and 1950s doctors jealously guarded medical knowledge, and only spoke in general terms about health in the media. Since the 1960s, this has changed at an accelerating pace. Today, newspapers, magazines and especially television are major carriers of information about health and illness. Moreover, where doctors once dominated such coverage, in a form which effectively maintained their 'hegemony' over medical information, other voices are now to be heard, including investigatory journalists, dissenting doctors, campaigners, academics (including, sometimes, sociologists), economists and health care managers. To this extent, 'medical dominance' of media coverage and of society can be seen to be waning (Bury and Gabe 1994).

More direct challenges to the doctor–patient relationship as the sole source of official medical information have stemmed from the related expansion of self-help groups, information systems (including, increasingly, the Internet), help lines, telephone counselling and the like. When these form part of campaigns about health issues or the actions of wider social movements, the central position of medicine, and thus of doctors, becomes even weaker. The growth of alternative medicine is also of relevance here, in part the result of dissatisfaction with the traditional doctor–patient relationship (R. Taylor 1984) and the 'attractiveness in . . . longer consultations and the holistic approach' to patients (Cant and Calnan 1991: 55; see also Saks 1992 and Sharma 1992). The nursing profession has also employed the idea of a more holistic view of illness, in an attempt to move away from a subservient position with regard to doctors, in the 'new nursing' approach (Witz 1994).

One of the most important and sustained challenges to medicine, as far as recent social movements are concerned, is, of course, the women's movement. Doyal (1994) makes the point that the most obvious area of conflict in feminist writing on modern medicine, as discussed earlier, has been in the area of reproductive health. Porter (1990) has commented, however, that despite considerable sociological and critical writing on this topic, evidence of a more shared view of care by doctors or of a less deferential view of care by women patients is sparse, and that feminist writing has not always represented the range of views held by women patients. Moreover, as Doyal notes, there is a tendency on the part of medicine, 'to ignore specifically or predominantly female problems unless they are connected with reproduction' (Doyal 1994: 146), and this has been repeated in feminist research. Note should be made, however, of the long-standing if problematic history of research, including social research, on women's psychological health (Busfield 1994). With respect to physical illness, Doyal cites the case of heart disease, where recent evidence suggests that ignoring symptoms, with delay in diagnosis and treatment by doctors (resulting from a bias towards regarding heart disease as a male disorder), has had serious implications for women patients. Recent evidence supports this contention (Healy 1991; Petticrew et al. 1993; Clarke et al. 1994).

Doyal, like Porter, notes that feminist challenges to patterns of treatment do not necessarily mean that changes in practice result. For example, when women general practitioners attempt to alter relationships this is likely to clash with the 'traditional relations of hierarchy' within health systems (Doyal 1994: 151). Despite these difficulties, Doyal argues that 'well women's clinics' have expanded rapidly, especially in the US, and have offered a new model of health care and doctor–patient relationships (see also Foster 1989). It might also be noted that attention to areas such as heart disease in women may signal an important change in outlook. Moreover, Doyal notes that some surgeons are 'beginning to pay attention' to the demand for greater autonomy in decision-making, especially in areas such as breast cancer (Doyal 1994: 151). While such challenges to medical dominance do not map on to existing doctor–patient relationships in a straightforward way, evidence in these areas suggests that a shift in the traditional patterns of care, as well as in public debate, may now be occurring.

Changes in medicine and the law are also important. Court cases involving doctors have occurred throughout modern medicine's history, but the scale of litigation and the willingness of patients in particular to turn to the law today – especially in Britain – marks a major increase in legal activity over the doctor–patient relationship.

In the US, a legalistic framework has long characterised the doctor–patient relationship. The number of claims brought by American patients has been consistently higher than in the UK (Dingwall *et al.* 1991). Though data on UK trends are difficult to interpret, it seems clear that there has been an increase in the frequency and severity of medical malpractice claims in the UK since the 1970s (Dingwall *et al.* 1991: 7). The increased fear of litigation, as well as its reality, is also reflected in the upsurge in costs for doctors' membership of the Medical Defence Union (which provides insurance cover for doctors), showing a year on year increase in subscription rates throughout the 1980s, particularly at the end of that decade (Dingwall *et al.* 1991: 19).

The authors of the report cited here make the point that it is difficult to judge the increased threat of malpractice litigation on doctors' behaviour. The possibility of a 'defensive medicine' developing has been widely discussed, especially in some specialties such as obstetrics. This could mean that the traditional doctor–patient relationship might give way to a situation in which the doctor departs from a normal or appropriate response, for example to ensure that tests or treatment are undertaken even when they are not deemed clinically necessary. The danger lies in the fact that such actions themselves may be hazardous, as doctors 'alter clinical practice in response to scanty or unfounded information' (Dingwall *et al.* 1991: 45).

For the present purposes, however, the most important feature of the changing legal context is the proposal that a more explicit 'market relationship' should exist between doctor and patient, in which their 'mutual liabilities' might be specified 'in a formal, individualised context' (Dingwall *et al.* 1991: 57). Following the work of Epstein (1976, 1977), Dingwall *et al.* argue that a formal *contractual* relationship would mean that doctors would be more careful about treating their patients. In turn, patients would be more careful in selecting their doctors and evaluating their performance. Though this formalised approach might have some attractions, Dingwall *et al.* note that the continuing 'asymmetrical' nature of the doctor–patient relationship makes this difficult to realise, especially for poor and chronically sick patients (Dingwall *et al.* 1991: 59).

Nevertheless, the fact that such arguments are being discussed seriously, especially, again, within the context of British medicine, is an indication of the extent of possible changes in the future patterns of the doctor–patient relationship. This view is reinforced when two other related changes currently under way are considered. The first of these concerns consumerism in health care. With the launch of the 'Patient's Charter' (DoH 1991) the Conservative government in Britain signalled an attempt to pursue a far more vigorous 'consumer-led' approach to health care than had been attempted hitherto. Medical sociologists such as Stacey argued in the 1970s that consumerism was not a relevant concept in the health care context (Stacey 1976), reflecting the long-held assumption that health care could not be regarded as a 'consumer good'. Today, 'charter standards', such as reducing waiting times in out-patient clinics and a general attempt to make the NHS more 'patient-oriented', have signalled a further shift in power from doctors to patients in a consumer-led direction. Nettleton and Harding (1994) have drawn attention to the growth in complaints made by 'protesting patients' to Family Health Service Authorities with respect to British general practitioners.

In addition, the 'managerial revolution' in the NHS has introduced a major change in organisation and outlook, again in an attempt to make the service more patient-oriented. As Hunter (1994) has noted, 'doctors are being compelled to define their practices and modes of operating in ways that many believe are undermining their professional values, and the ability to act in accordance with such values' (Hunter 1994: 1). However, even though an 'ascendant management' may be able to alter the overall balance of power decisively away from doctors, Hunter argues that the standing of doctors 'among the public' remains high, and 'they will continue to possess considerable power to contain counter-vailing forces' (Hunter 1994: 19). Elston has also noted that reductions in the 'political' or 'economic autonomy' of doctors do not add up to a 'major waning' of 'clinical autonomy' (Elston 1991: 83; see also, on general practice, Calnan and Gabe 1991: 158). Challenges by other professional groups such as nurses, as noted earlier, may also be resisted (Witz 1994: 34). Though this suggests that changes in doctor–patient or inter-professional relationships are not likely to proceed in a straight line, it is equally evident that they will become the site of continuing and complex processes in the future.

Evaluation and the doctor–patient relationship

Part of the new health care agenda which has grown up alongside managerialism and professional change concerns the increasing role for research and evidence in health care practice. This constitutes the last area of change to be considered here.

To stay with Hunter's analysis for a moment, this notes that the British government's emphasis on research and development within the NHS 'should in theory provide ammunition, in the form of empirical evidence concerning medical treatments and their effectiveness, for managers to challenge doctors' (Hunter 1994: 20). Whether this will turn out to be an important political device it is too early to say. Doctors have already seen the possibilities of managerially led research on evaluation, especially in such areas as the 'outcomes' of treatment, 'evidence-based health care' and patient satisfaction with care. They too are now pursuing such research, partly in order to keep ahead of the game.

The potential for such research findings to affect the doctor–patient relationship directly may not be immediately obvious, but if taken alongside the other developments discussed above their impact could be significant. Evidence on variations in outcomes, especially comparisons of doctors using the same treatment modalities, could become powerful sources of information for patients. This will add to already available material on waiting lists and other organisational aspects of the health care system. The British consumer group, the College of Health, for example, provides routine information about various features of NHS performance, and the Department of Health in Britain now issues a 'league table' on the performance of hospitals, though at present excluding data on clinical outcomes. Other organisations aimed at informing patients about aspects of clinical treatment for specific disorders (e.g. cancer) have also grown rapidly in recent years.

In such a context, evaluative research may not simply be a long-term feature of the managerial challenge to medicine, but may be assimilated more widely by patients themselves. This will set up a new set of strains in the doctor–patient relationship. It is likely to exacerbate the situation described earlier, in which conflict arises from the desire of doctors to have informed patients while at the same keeping demand for care, and medical knowledge about disease, under their control. Researching outcomes is likely to encourage a more 'contractual' outlook among patients, who may want their doctors to inform them in detail about the risks and benefits of treatment, where trust in the doctor's judgement once held sway. While some practitioners may welcome such developments, others may be resistant.

CONCLUDING COMMENT

The situation described above poses one of the main dilemmas for medical sociology and the contemporary study of the doctor–patient relationship. The first part of this chapter examined models of the doctor–patient relationship that were relevant to a period in which doctors held centre stage in the health care system. Much sociological work was preoccupied in revealing the extent and effects of medical power and 'dominance'. Today, however, sociologists are increasingly involved in studying the 'patient's viewpoint', researching both clinical and quality of life outcomes, as well as patient satisfaction, as part of the evaluative context described above. There is now a growing literature on measuring health and disease outcomes (Bowling 1991, 1995) and on the problems in doing so (Donovan *et al.* 1993; Fitzpatrick and Albrecht 1994), as well as extended discussions of patient satisfaction measures and their limitations (e.g. Carr-Hill 1992).

While this work is likely to remain an important field of study for medical sociologists, there is a danger of the incorporation of researchers as well as clinicians into a research agenda almost entirely set by governments and managers. Extensive research on patient satisfaction, for example, may paradoxically blunt the edge of a critical analysis by endlessly surveying patients' views with little or no demonstrable effect. It will be remembered that Stimson and Webb warned against reductionist views of the complex processes that go to make up the doctor–patient relationship. Hospitals and general practices may gather large quantities of simplistic data – on 'customer feedback' through 'eliciting standardised replies' (Long 1994: 178) – in order to show how effective or responsive they are, while services may be deteriorating 'on the ground'. While 'evidence-based health care' is an important development, it may be used to ration services rather than improve them.

In addition, such research may be less than valuable for older patients and others for whom clear-cut 'outcomes' are not always relevant. In such circumstances, patients may come to see doctors' 'clinical judgement' as an important defence of their needs against managerialism, and indeed against research evidence that denies them treatment. A contractual model based on managerial principles runs the risk of patients losing power rather than gaining it, as Freidson has argued (Freidson 1988: 387). Somewhat ironically, Freidson also argues that clinical autonomy may now act as a bulwark against the negative effects of 'official' (i.e. managerial) medicine and an over-concern with efficiency. Doctors may now be the best allies of patients, mediating between them 'and the formal system' (Freidson 1988: 401).

Within the shifting scene that is today's health care system, a narrowing of the focus in 'official' research to a concern only with measuring outcomes and patient satisfaction would be a step backwards. Much evaluation research is concerned with documenting practice with the laudable aim of improving services, but without asking fundamental research questions about patients' experiences. Public debate about the nature of the doctor–patient and other health care interactions may suffer as a result. This is the case even where such developments are linked with the growth in applied research opportunities. The new research agenda needs to continue to include the critical themes of earlier interpretive medical sociology research on the doctor–patient relationship, if the patient's viewpoint is to be heard clearly in the future. Recent interest in the role of qualitative methods in health services research (Pope and Mays 1995) suggests, however, that the research agenda may develop in a way that can keep genuine debate as well as the production of useful information alive.

Chapter 4

Chronic illness and disability

INTRODUCTION

Some years ago Herbert Blumer, the American sociologist, made the point that much sociological research tackles problems 'in the wake of societal recognition' (Blumer 1971: 299). It certainly seems clear that issues which have already been identified by public bodies are more likely to provide opportunities for (funded) research than those that have not. Research in medical sociology is no exception. It has both benefited and suffered from dealing with problems already identified as social concerns and reflected in health policy and medical agendas. The massive rise in research on HIV/AIDS in the 1980s and 1990s is an obvious case in point. It has been argued elsewhere in this book that the growth of medical sociology has frequently been influenced by the fortunes and problems of specific areas of medicine, such as public health and general practice.

The sociological study of chronic illness tells a similar story. With the rise in importance of chronic illness in post-Second World War industrial societies, social concerns about its consequences have grown, and some areas of medicine have found themselves vulnerable to identity crises in a situation where clinical interventions have been unable to deliver cures. In contrast with the optimism that swept surgery, especially transplant surgery, in the 1970s, the care of the chronically ill has been less rewarding for both patient and doctor alike, and certainly less dramatic. Not only this, but many of the problems faced by patients with chronic disorders have been unavoidably social in nature, and specialists responsible for their care have looked outside of the medical arena for help in meeting the challenges they pose. It is this which helps explain why sociological work on chronic illness and disability has been far more prominent than work on the experience of surgery and acute medicine, where, rightly or wrongly, clinicians have been more confident about their activities.

Sociologists have thus been 'invited in' to work on chronic illness, as they have been in areas such as inequalities and the doctor–patient relationship. Behind these developments, however, lie changes of a more profound nature in the patterns of health and illness and in the wider culture, creating fertile ground for greater public as well as medical and sociological recognition. The importance of contemporary morbidity and mortality patterns and, especially, their relationship with changing demographic profiles in modern societies is central to an overall grasp of the place of chronic illness in social life. The long-term reduction in mortality rates (along with the secular decline in fertility) has meant that modern societies have undergone a powerful 'demographic transition' towards an older population structure, and this has become a global trend, to a greater or lesser degree (Bury 1992a). In turn, illnesses associated with later life have become more prominent than they were in the past, as, for the first time, old age has become 'commonplace' (Arie 1988). As a result of these changes in longevity and improved survival, the examination of health disorders at different points in the life course have become a major source of interest for medical sociologists.

At the cultural level the study of chronic illness touches on equally important issues. With the demographic transition has come a 'cultural transition'. In many modern societies a situation has developed where the constraints of life-threatening disease, early death and insecurity have given way to a more predictable life course, in the context of a relatively safe social and physical environment. As a result, a more open and plural 'life world' has developed with an emphasis on life planning and self-identity as active and feasible 'projects' (Berger *et al.* 1974). Under these conditions control and display of 'normal appearances' in everyday life, to use Goffman's term, has come to the fore (Goffman 1971). Central to this has been the contention that 'control of the body is integral to the very nature of agency and of being accepted (trusted) by others as competent' (Giddens 1991: 57). Indeed, the need to display 'cultural competence' in a variety of different ways has become a defining characteristic of modern society (Hirst and Woolley 1982).

Disability and illness which interfere with claims to 'competence' therefore touch on critical cultural and moral frameworks which link the body, self and society (see also chapter 6). As will be seen below, the study of chronic illness has therefore been an important way of examining aspects of identity, social interaction, the experience of stigma and the body in late modern society, and provides an important window on the relationship between agency and structure. Sociological interest has thus been concerned not only with the documentation of the problems people face, but also with the actions they take to mitigate the threat which illness entails. This also brings into the picture, once again, relationships between lay and professional modes of action and thought.

In all these ways the study of chronic illness and disability can be seen to go to the heart of contemporary social and cultural developments. Against this backdrop, the chapter proceeds along the following lines. First, it fills out, in somewhat more detail, the changing patterns of health and illness mentioned above. In particular, it describes the relationship between chronic illness and disability as it has emerged in modern societies. Second, the chapter discusses the emergence of a 'socio-medical' model of chronic illness and disability, which has provided the framework for collaboration between public health doctors, medical specialists and medical sociologists that took place in the 1970s and 1980s. Third, the main lines of more independent sociological research on chronic illness are examined, with particular reference to an interpretive framework within which patients' experiences and actions have been situated. Finally, future directions of research on chronic illness are discussed within a changing context which is affecting both the researched and the researcher. Here, the development of a more 'contestable' culture will be identified, with particular respect to the rise of the 'disability movement' and its impact on the future agenda for sociological work.

CHANGING PATTERNS OF HEALTH AND ILLNESS

If the single most important change in the pattern of health and illness in modern times were to be identified, it would surely be the rise and fall of the infections. It is difficult today, despite the occurrence of HIV/AIDS, to grasp the magnitude of the impact of the infections on industrial societies in the past. Public opinion in modern societies is still made aware of the continuing relevance of infections to the health of people in developing countries. And the possible recurrence of such disease, if deteriorating social conditions permit, eloquently argued by Dubos in the 1960s (Dubos 1960) and by others since (e.g. Evans 1987), is often mentioned in news reporting. But the collective memory and personal experience of diseases such as cholera, typhus, rheumatic fever and diphtheria have largely disappeared in Western societies, though their names echo down the years. Other conditions such as smallpox remain only a name, as a result of their complete elimination from human populations.

Yet in the nineteenth and well into the twentieth century, infections such as cholera and tuberculosis (TB) were the scourge of many communities throughout the modern world. It has been recently argued that in the early nineteenth century 'it is likely that one in four deaths in the cities of Europe was attributable to consumption', and in the middle of the century 100,000 deaths per annum in England and Wales alone were being recorded (Webster 1994: 38). Webster goes on to say that even in '1900 medical experts regarded TB as the greatest single threat to health' (ibid.). Despite McKeown's (1976) argument that medical care played only a minor role in reducing the impact of infections such as TB, and Szreter's subsequent critique emphasising more strongly the role of public health measures (Szreter 1988), it was only through the combination of improving social conditions and effective treatment after 1945 that conditions such as TB were effectively suppressed. Deaths from respiratory tuberculosis declined by no less than 98 per cent between 1946 and 1982 (Wells 1984: 9).

Earlier, the infections were particularly important as causes of morbidity and mortality in early life, either in infancy or in early adult years. This resulted in a dramatic effect on average life expectancy at birth in the first part of the twentieth century. In Britain in 1901, life expectancy at birth was only 45.5 years for men and 49 for women (CSO 1995). With the progressive reduction in the burden of infectious disease at the early stages of the life course, together with a reduction in the numbers of children being born, the proportion of the population living into middle and later life increased. Not only has the average life expectancy at birth improved, therefore, standing today at nearly 80 for women and 74 for men (CSO 1995), but the population structure as a whole has become considerably older. Today some 16 per cent of the population is now over the retirement age (compared with 11 per cent in 1951) and as life expectancy has improved in later years, as well as in early life, the very old have increased as a proportion of all elderly people (Alderson 1988; Jefferys and Thane 1989).

The effects of the reduction of infectious diseases such as TB have not, of course, been confined to improvement in survival. While the control of disease has been pursued as a positive, almost self-evident social goal, unintended consequences have also been produced. As the infections have waned, so degenerative health disorders, associated with later life, have grown. Today, heart disease is the largest single cause of death, followed by cancer, both major sources of disability. Other disorders such as stroke, arthritis and Parkinson's disease have become more prominent, associated as they are with later life. As will be discussed in more detail below, this has led, again in McKeown's (1976) terms, to a shift in concern from cure to care, and in some respects, therefore, from the importance of medical services to social welfare.

In the context of a discussion of chronic illness, however, it is important not to overstate the contrast between infectious disease and non-infectious disease. There are at least two reasons to be cautious in this respect. First, many of the features of chronic illness which are of concern today, especially the consequences of disorders with a long and uncertain duration, were first noticed in infectious conditions such as TB. The need for long-term care was already apparent in this disorder from the earliest days, and interestingly one of the first studies of the experience of chronic illness was carried out by a sociologist suffering from it (Roth 1963). In this study Roth drew attention to the important matter of the *temporal dimension* of chronic illness ('chronic' from the Greek *khronos*, meaning time) and the uncertainty which characterises many of the actions both patients and professionals face in its management? Roth documented in particular the ways in which negotiating release from long-stay hospitals, for example, were social in character, based on conventional 'timetables' for the illness, rather than being strictly dictated by clinical evidence of cure.

Second, as effective medical treatments have improved, particularly in recent years, the boundary between medical and social care in chronic illness has become weaker (Gerhardt 1990; Bury 1994b). Though some forms of medical care for chronic disorders have remained relatively static over the years, others have not. Even for those that pose the most intractable problems, such as stroke and arthritis, services offering medical care, rehabilitation, physiotherapy and speech therapy have undergone large-scale expansion.

Specialist medical treatment for older patients, almost unheard of in Britain where widespread geriatric care was favoured instead, is also now undergoing considerable change (Jennett 1988: 179–180). The surgical treatment of disorders such as renal failure, hip replacement and especially heart disease and cancer in older people is changing fast, and has been associated with the decline in importance of geriatrics. While the latter offered a 'safety net' for the elderly in social as well as medical terms, community care is now supposed to meet the social needs of the elderly.

The question of age is also associated with another issue to be discussed in this chapter, namely the relationship between chronic illness and disability. As Taylor pointed out some twenty years ago, 'in numerical terms those who become disabled before middle life form only a small proportion of the total number' (D. Taylor 1977: 8). In the first years of life conditions such as hydrocephalus and cerebral palsy (including what used to be called spasticity) are the main causes of disability, followed by road and sports accidents in later childhood and early adulthood (Oliver et al. 1988). In the past, war and industrial injury dominated disability in adult life and the rehabilitation services set up to deal with it. Far more numerous today, however, even when the degree of severity is taken into account, is the disabling impact of chronic illness in later life (Martin et al. 1988). Although, of course, the stage of the life course at which disability begins has important implications for the amount and duration of care needed, the majority of those with disabilities today are older people with chronic illnesses. The implications of these changes for research in the field will be touched upon at various points in this chapter.

For the present, however, the point needs to be underlined that the study of chronic illness and disability goes to the heart of the development of contemporary society, and not only its demographic structure. As Stone (1984) has pointed out in the British context and Albrecht in the US (Albrecht 1992), modern social structures and especially their welfare institutions revolve round responses to disability and chronic illness. Decisions concerning financial and legal compensation, social security payments and many other matters hinge on the ability of modern social systems to conceptualise, monitor and effect surveillance over a host of chronic illnesses and disabilities. It might be added that the associated features of an ageing population are equally at the centre of key decisions about patterns of health care and public expenditure.

These go far beyond the confines of the clinic or home. The public health, economic and, indeed, political dimensions of chronic illness, give it an importance which its apparently marginalised medical status may disguise.

THE SOCIO-MEDICAL MODEL OF DISABLING ILLNESS

Until recently, the main aims of public health and epidemiology have been with the mapping of patterns of disease and with *disease surveillance*. Even today, despite the overall decline of the infections, outbreaks of such disease continue to present challenges to the public health services, as the examples of salmonella and legionnella in the 1980s testified. Mention has already been made of HIV/AIDS, which has promoted a world-wide epidemiological response. One of the objectives of such activity has traditionally been to identify the causes of infection and therefore the possible source of preventive action. Every student of public health has been told the story of the Broad Street pump in London's Soho. There, in 1854, John Simon, the famous Victorian surgeon turned public health doctor, used careful analysis of death rates by geographical area to trace an outbreak of cholera to contaminated water supplied by one pump (Bynum 1994: 79). By removing the handle of the pump the outbreak was halted. The moral of the story is that even if the actual aetiological agent is not fully understood (as was the case with cholera) careful analysis of disease patterns can lead to the identification and implementation of preventive measures. For this reason, mortality data have preoccupied epidemiologists, and continue to do so despite their limitations.

Paradoxically, however, as mortality data have been better understood they have become less relevant as measures of public health (Patrick 1986; see also chapter 2). This is not only because diseases associated with later life are likely to result in long-term illness rather than death, but also because their aetiological picture is far more complex than that of the infections. Though evidence of 'risk factors' for disorders such as cancer and heart disease have received considerable attention, the origins of conditions such as arthritis, Parkinson's disease and even stroke remain largely a mystery. Screening aimed at preventing these diseases is rarely appropriate, except, perhaps, with such factors as blood pressure and stroke prevention. Moreover, in a period of falling death rates, the preoccupation with mortality has seemed increasingly problematic in public health circles, especially as calls for health services to adopt more positive health promotion strategies have increased. As has been seen in chapter 1, maintaining health as much as preventing life-threatening disease has become the order of the day.

For these reasons, attention in both the US and Britain has slowly turned to the *consequences* of disease rather than its cause. In the US sociologists with strong public health links debated in the 1960s whether social conditions were implicated in the occurrence of chronic disorders or, more importantly, with their consequences. In an exchange between Kadushin (1966) and Mechanic (1968) much of the subsequent debate about general health inequalities was rehearsed. Kadushin maintained that, in post-war American society, there was not a significant relationship between social class and the occurrence of chronic illness, though 'social drift' might be at work leading to downward social mobility among the chronically ill. Mechanic, on the other hand, pointed to the possible effects of poverty on the occurrence of illness as well as the additional costs of the consequences of living with disability, arguing that 'disease affects earnings and work status' (Mechanic 1968: 262). Then, in 1973, Conover renewed the debate in the US by publishing a new analysis of the original data used by Kadushin. This showed that structural factors could be identified as being strongly correlated with patterns of onset of chronic illness, as Mechanic had suggested (Conover 1973).

In Britain, research on the social dimensions of chronic illness (especially their consequences) also began in the 1960s, though, it has to be said, within a less explicit sociological framework. For example, collaboration between the public health oriented rehabilitation specialist Michael Warren and the sociologist Margot Jefferys focused on the assessment of motor impairment in prevalence studies of disabling illness (Jefferys *et al.* 1969). As Patrick has subsequently pointed out, such work was linked to estimating medical need and the possibility of developing secondary preventive strategies, that is, preventing deterioration rather than initial onset (Patrick and Peach 1989: 21). This early work of Jefferys and others culminated in the national study *Handicapped and Impaired in Great Britain* carried out by Amelia Harris and published in 1971 (Harris *et al.* 1971). This showed, for the first time, the extent of impairment in Britain, and suggested that just under 4 per cent of the population aged 16 to 64 and just under 28 per cent of the population over the age of 65 were suffering from some form of impairment. Importantly, gender differences were also noted, with twice the level of impairment in women compared with men. Comparable prevalence studies were carried out in the US at this time (Patrick and Peach 1989: 22).

Subsequently, in Britain, Wood and his colleagues sought to clarify the terminology that was being used in this research, especially in the light of confusing usage even in the Harris survey, where different terms (e.g. 'impairment' and 'handicap') were sometimes used synonymously. In 1980 the World Health Organisation published the results of this work in the form of the *International Classification of Impairments, Disabilities and Handicaps* (ICIDH) which provided more consistent definitions (WHO 1980). In this classification, *impairment* referred to abnormality in the structure of the functioning of the body, whether through disease or trauma, *disability* referred to activity restriction and the inability to perform everyday tasks, especially those associated with self-care, and *handicap* referred to the social disadvantage that could be associated with either impairment or disability. The last term was particularly emphasised as a means of underlining material and social needs created by the consequences of chronic illness (Bury 1979).

The widespread use of this schema helped both to develop the socio-medical model that earlier work had been building and to provide the basis for considerable debate and research development in the years that followed. Community-based studies such as that in Lambeth, south London, mentioned above (Patrick and Peach 1989) also explored the prevalence of impairment and the health care and rehabilitation needs in disability. In recent years the schema has also been employed to map social aspects of handicap, such as material hardship and the role of social support. This kind of research has thus helped to examine the mediating relationship between the various planes of experience that the WHO schema had described (Patrick and Peach 1989; Harwood *et al.* 1994).

National and local studies underlined, in the British context, the economic dimensions of disability and the hardship experienced by many, particularly in a period of growing recession. Though the Harris survey had been associated with the passing of the 1970 Chronically Sick and Disabled Persons Act, which for the first time obliged local authorities in Britain to estimate and meet the needs of the disabled, various research findings reinforced the view, held by Mechanic in the earlier US work, that it was in financial hardship that the consequences of disability were most obviously seen.

Townsend's compendious work on *Poverty in the United Kingdom* gave additional weight to the link between disability and inequality in these terms (Townsend 1979).

However, though the socio-medical model has provided the grounds for identifying and drawing attention to the various needs of the chronically sick and disabled, many problems have remained. At the research level, it has long been recognised that the category of disability, despite clarification in the WHO schema, is 'relational' in character; where infectious disease could be defined in categorical terms and had a defining hallmark (e.g. either the tubercule bacillus was present or it was absent), disability involved judgements of degree and context. It was pointed out that the term 'disability' was conceptually 'slippery' and difficult to pin down (Topliss 1979) and that the dividing line between impairment, disability and handicap was difficult to operationalise, important though these distinctions were (Bury 1987).

At the political level, though the consequences of disability were being more widely appreciated during the 1970s, financial compensation and an increased role for disabled people to influence the agenda lagged behind. In part this arose from the continuing role that medicine played, within administrative circles, in defining disability and adjudicating applications for benefits. In order to tackle this problem and provide estimates of disability based on a more systematic approach, a new national study was commissioned by the British Office of Population Censuses and Surveys (OPCS) in 1984, and several surveys, including one on children, were carried out between 1985 and 1988. The main purpose of this new initiative was to inform a review of social security in the disability field and pave the way for such benefits to be based less on medical assessment. This has been achieved with the advent of the Disability Living Allowance and the Disability Working Allowance (Bury 1996a).

Of importance to the present discussion is the fact that the OPCS undertook to develop disability assessments which would be sensitive to the difficulties encountered in earlier work. By combining judgements of professionals, researchers and disabled people themselves (through close co-operation with organisations such as the Royal National Institute for the Blind and the Disability Alliance) and by using the basic definition of disability as laid down in the WHO classification, the OPCS was able to operationalise a new, more sociologically informed and contextualised approach.

Scales were developed in key areas of disability, ranging from problems with locomotion through seeing, hearing and personal care to difficulties with communication (Martin *et al.* 1988: 10). By focusing directly on the nature and impact of disability (but not on impairment) this approach shifted the centre of gravity of the socio-medical model away from the clinic and towards a more systematic approach to disability in everyday life.

For the present purpose, two main findings are of note. First, the association of disability with age was once again confirmed. The survey showed that of six million people living in Great Britain with at least one form of disability, based on the relatively low threshold used in the survey, almost 70 per cent of disabled adults were aged 60 and over, and nearly half were aged 70 and over (Martin *et al.* 1988: 27). The very old emerge as those most likely to be affected, with 63 per cent of women and 53 per cent of men over the age of 75 being disabled. When severity is taken into account, the very old predominate, with 64 per cent of adults in the two highest categories aged 70 or over and 41 per cent aged 80 or over (ibid.). Given that women significantly outnumber men at this age, the gender imbalance in chronic illness is clearly of note. The significance of some of these findings will be returned to later in the chapter.

The predominance of chronic illness as the cause of disability is also of note in the OPCS study. Many of the disorders associated with later life, especially arthritis and hearing loss (the former helping to explain much of the gender difference in disability rates), were the most frequent causes of disability. This underlined the long-term trend, noted earlier, away from disabilities caused by trauma and medical conditions in early life towards those associated with illness in later life. Though not all forms of disability are caused by chronic illness, most are.

Important though this study was in developing and improving the picture available from the earlier Harris study, the role of chronic illness in the findings does expose some of the tensions found in this area of work. For no matter how justifiable the attempt to reduce the role of medical definitions and adjudication, a full picture of disability inevitably exposes its disease or health disorder dimensions. For those experiencing disability, therefore, different dimensions are relevant, variously articulating health and social needs. Some people with stable disabilities not involving illness may regard the role of health care as marginal to their experience. For others, especially those suffering from fluctuating or degenerative chronic illness, health care and social welfare may be needed in different ways and at different times.

This issue of the wide variation in experience has been associated, for sociologists at least, with a growing concern with the *meaning* of disability and not simply its definition or prevalence. Within the body of work on the socio-medical model, therefore, a more independent sociological voice began to emerge, despite the medical and policy agendas which had dominated the field until then. This new approach began to apply more explicitly sociological concepts to the area. In Britain, Mildred Blaxter's book *The Meaning of Disability* (Blaxter 1976) and in the US Strauss's book, *Chronic Illness and the Quality of Life* (Strauss 1975) captured the spirit of these concerns. Since that time more clearly focused sociological work on chronic illness and disability has begun to emerge.

THE SOCIOLOGY OF CHRONIC ILLNESS AND DISABILITY

Despite its avowed intent to develop a sociological perspective, Strauss's book (Strauss 1975) began by making a link between sociological concern with chronic illness and its significance in public health terms. The growing importance of chronic illness within the American population was noted in a long introductory essay, as was the need for more focused study. Strauss particularly emphasised the need to document the impact of chronic illness on daily life. The rest of the book comprised a series of condition-specific studies, employing qualitative methods in order to address the experiences of patients and their families directly. However, a paradox was potentially involved here, as the disease categories used to identify patient groups were precisely part of the problem to be investigated. If the meaning of illness was to be elucidated, then the role of medical care and its 'labelling' was bound to be part of the story. However, the basic premise of this work, and much that followed it, was that the disorders in question were real sources of pain and suffering and had definite social consequences. Condition-specific empirical work actually underlined the importance of disease categories to lay people at certain points in their 'illness trajectory', especially in being able to identify and name the source of the threat being faced. This observation was often made despite the fact that medical sociologists elsewhere were arguing strongly about the presence of medical dominance and the 'medicalisation of life' (see chapter 1).

Having said this, most of the substantive chapters of Strauss's book were taken up by accounts of the *interactional difficulties* encountered by people living with disabling illness. Wiener's study of rheumatoid arthritis and Fagerhaugh's study of respiratory illness, for example, showed patients negotiating their way through a social terrain in which everyday interaction had been spoiled (Wiener 1975; Fagerhaugh 1975). Wiener's respondents described how they attempted to 'pass for normal' and disguise their arthritic symptoms, so as to avoid negative and stigmatising responses. A delicate 'balancing of decisions' was employed in attempts to maintain normal life, where the expenditure of effort needed to be constantly set against the consequences (Wiener 1975: 80). Fagerhaugh showed how patients with respiratory symptoms spent a great deal of time managing symptoms of breathlessness and lack of oxygen. Again, the intrusion of these symptoms on the fabric and quality of everyday life was emphasised, as were the attempts to manage it. The themes of maintaining a sense of order, self-identity and social interaction under conditions of considerable strain were evident. These studies exemplified a set of more theoretical considerations in micro sociology, concerning 'negotiated order' in a changing culture and 'grounded theory', building up sociological categories from first-hand accounts and observations, with which Strauss, following Goffman, was concerned (Glaser and Strauss 1965, 1967).

In Britain, meanwhile, Blaxter's book *The Meaning of Disability* was drawing on a somewhat broader framework in mapping out a sociological view of chronic illness and its consequences. Blaxter interviewed 100 patients during the year after discharge from a Scottish hospital, following treatment for a variety of chronic medical conditions. Unlike Strauss's colleagues, Blaxter was less interested in documenting the detail of interactional difficulties than in establishing the various 'problems' patients and their families faced during the year in question. These ranged from continuing medical troubles and problems with housing to wider social difficulties. However, in line with Strauss and Glaser, it was these last that Blaxter found to be the most intractable.

Blaxter showed that although medical care was important to patients in chronic illness, the main issues had to be faced outside of its orbit. For the majority of patients and their families, unresolved problems of maintaining social relationships, both in the home and outside, were most important at the end of the year in question. Blaxter also showed that official agencies could exacerbate these difficulties as well as help to tackle them. In particular, she drew attention to the conflicting definitions of problems faced by chronically ill patients, with professional agencies (e.g. health services and social services) operating with different assumptions. Bureaucratic procedures often confounded patients' efforts to respond. Blaxter therefore used her survey to draw attention to the policy implications of the meaning of disability, and called for more coherence in the care of and social policy response to the chronically ill.

These two themes, interactional difficulties and the nature of professional responses to chronic illness, have run through most subsequent medical sociology work. An inductive approach, using qualitative methods within an interpretive framework, has dominated most sociological studies of chronic illness (Gerhardt 1989). Whilst interactionism and a concern with 'everyday life' has been criticised in mainstream sociology for its lack of attention to *social hierarchy* and the rules and resources that influence life in modern societies (Mouzelis 1991), this seems only partly true in the study of chronic illness in medical sociology. Attention to the routine encounters between patients and agents of health and welfare systems, as well as to the social and material consequences of illness, has made the question of 'rules and resources' central to at least some of its depictions of experience. Moreover, an emphasis on the *active* response to chronic illness has suggested ways in which agency and structure can be examined in medical sociology.

Emerging from this work, three aspects of the experience of and response to chronic illness may be distinguished. First is the *biographical disruption* brought about by such illness and the initial attempts to deal with the uncertainty it brings; second is the *impact of treatment* on everyday life, where this is relevant; and third is the long-term *adaptation and management* of illness and disability which is undertaken as people respond and try to reconstruct normal life. Though some researchers, especially those following the approach of Strauss, may see these aspects of experience in terms of stages or as part of an illness trajectory across the life course, the suggested predictability may be overstated. In contrast, the *emergent* quality of experience is emphasised here, and thus the analytic rather than the sequential or predictive value of the approach.

Biographical disruption

Though illness may be expected to occur at some point in most people's lives, it was argued above that modern cultures are premised on a general expectation of long life and of health. As Parsons noted, values such as activism and achievement orientation require an optimum level of health in society (Parsons 1958) and an expectation of it at the individual level (Parsons 1978: 72). The expression of this in the association between a sense of control and health in lay thought (Crawford 1984) has already been noted in the earlier discussion of lay beliefs, as has the increased emphasis on health in general (chapter 1).

The onset of illness, especially that which is not evidently self-limiting, fractures this social and cultural fabric, exposing the individual to threats to self-identity and a potentially damaging loss of control. The term *biographical disruption* was coined to give expression to these processes (Bury 1982, 1991). Treating chronic illness as a disruptive event in this way allows for its meaning to be situated in a temporal and life-course context. Changes in the body and the onset of symptoms simultaneously involve an alteration in the person's life situation and social relationships. Corbin and Strauss (1988) have used the term 'biographical body conceptions' (BBCs) in their depiction of the processes involved.

Two types of meaning can be seen to be involved in the onset of chronic illness (Bury 1988). The first of these concerns the *consequences* that the onset and persistence of symptoms have for people at the practical and social level. Condition-specific studies of disorders such as multiple sclerosis (I. Robinson 1988), diabetes (Kelleher 1988) and chronic respiratory disorder (S. Williams 1993) have shown how symptoms disrupt the normal flow of everyday life and introduce a growing sense of uncertainty into it. At this level the meaning of illness often involves a growing awareness of its potentially disabling effects, as self-care activities and other forms of daily life, whether at work or in the home, become problematic. Preoccupation with the management of symptoms and attempts to limit their practical consequences result.

The second set of concerns and meanings revolves round the *significance* of illness. Whilst the disabling effects of chronic illness often have common features (for example, the measurable limitations they place on task performance), the deeper significance of a disorder for a person's identity may be more specific. This concerns the symbolic significance disease, disability and illness have within segments of modern cultures, the metaphorical roles they play in everyday discourse and the attendant expectations people have of them. The onset of epilepsy, for example, involves dealing with the meaning of the term as well as the illness, against an historical backdrop of fear and apprehension, though this may now be waning to some extent (Schneider and Conrad 1983; Scambler and Hopkins 1988). Similarly in arthritis, sufferers, especially women, may attempt to disguise their symptoms, even from relatives, partly because of images of disfigurement and deformity associated with the diagnosis, and the thought that they may be seen as ageing prematurely (Singer 1974). In one study, respondents' husbands who were themselves suffering from conditions such as heart disease expressed far less inhibition in interview settings, because of the almost positive associations this has with overwork and stress (Bury 1988). Other research on conditions such as cancer of the bowel (Macdonald 1988) has described the debilitating effect of stigma that has to be managed alongside the effects of symptoms themselves.

As people begin to face up to the consequences of long-term illness and disability, various kinds of processes come into play. Biographical disruption can be mitigated in at least two ways: efforts may be made to construct a reasonable level of *explanation* for the illness and to establish its *legitimacy* in the person's life. While people may not always need to answer the questions 'Why me?' or 'Why now?' beloved of anthropologists (fatalism, for example, might dictate 'Why not me?'), the need for a form of 'repair' to the fabric of the person's life has been noted in a number of empirical studies. Again, work on arthritis serves to illustrate the point. In interviews reported by G. Williams (1984; G. Williams *et al.* 1996) individuals were found to be concerned with establishing a form of 'narrative reconstruction' of events leading up to and through the illness, in order to reduce its threat to the everyday meanings that had hitherto prevailed.

Linked to this process is the idea of legitimation. In the general sociological literature this denotes the process through which (political) authority is made credible (Bury 1991: 456). In the context of illness and biographical disruption, legitimation refers to the attempts by people to establish the place of a disabling illness within an altered daily life and within the web of social relationships in which the person's life may be enmeshed. Effort, at this level, is aimed at sustaining claims to 'cultural competence' and personal authority in the face of threat. This might involve working on close or 'proximate' relationships in which the presence of the illness will have to be reconciled, including intimate forms of interaction. It will also mean establishing an altered identity in more distant forms of social contact. Thus private and public dimensions of living with the illness must be fashioned to reduce its disruptive effects.

The impact of treatment and health care

In the situation described above, people are likely to approach health services with ambivalent feelings. As part of the 'resources' available to meet disruption through illness, health care systems offer reassurance at a time of apprehension and anxiety. On the other hand they open up concerns about the long-term nature of the disorder. Such contact also involves coming to grips with treatment regimens and medical interventions, and with the bureaucracies from which they emanate. The process of official diagnosis and labelling, from this viewpoint, may be regarded with relief as threatening events are brought under a degree of control, but this is not always a straightforward matter. Comaroff and Maguire (1981), reporting on a study of childhood leukaemia, found that modern medical knowledge of the condition helped reduce uncertainty for parents, but at the same time revealed more of what was not known. The transformation of fatal diseases into chronic ones may create unintended consequences of this kind, which then have to be handled by both professionals and patients alike. At times, patients and their relatives may experience this as a form of 'medical merry go round' (I. Robinson 1988) as searches are made for information and treatment that make sense and can be incorporated into a restructured social world and workable illness narratives. Sociological work has found, however, that as time passes the 'medical merry go round' slows down. The absorption of information about the illness and its treatment, together with the ritualised nature of medical encounters, increases the person's confidence. In Giddens' terminology, 're-skilling' occurs, offsetting the 'de-skilling' and powerlessness that encounters with experts may initially involve (Giddens 1991). Patients may become 'experts' themselves, about both the condition and its treatment, 'reading up' on them, swapping notes with other patients and gleaning further information from the media or relevant organisations. However, this may make further contacts with professionals such as general practitioners difficult, as the patient comes to doubt the doctor's level of expertise. GPs, of course, may recognise this process and may try to work with the patient in a form of 'meeting between experts' (Tuckett *et al.* 1985 – see chapter 3).

This process also suggests that patients are not only concerned with the 'affective' side of the doctor–patient relationship, but actively negotiate over technical information about the condition and its management. Fine judgements ensue about the costs and benefits (social as much as economic) of treatment, especially drug regimens. Studies have shown that in conditions such as multiple sclerosis and arthritis, patients become knowledgeable about the symptom-reducing effects of steroids and other anti-inflammatory drugs and about differing opinions of their side-effects. A 'careful pattern of experimentation' may be undertaken in deciding such matters (I. Robinson 1988: 86). The same study suggested that 'pooling expertise' of patient and practitioner is a more useful way forward than the medical preoccupation with 'patient compliance' (ibid.).

As treatment regimens become established, lay people monitor their impact and their interaction with the original disorder. Williams in his recent study of respiratory illness outlines several criteria which patients use in order to evaluate their medical regimens as time progresses (S. Williams 1993). These are: first, the degree of symptomatic or subjective relief that the treatment offers; second, the extent to which it helps to facilitate independence of activity in everyday life, that is, reduce disability in terms of 'activities of daily living'; third, the risks and acceptability of any perceived side-effects of the treatment; fourth, the amount of time, difficulty and restriction treatment involves, and fifth, the degree of intrusiveness or embarrassment that maintaining a regimen involves. Importantly, as with illness and disability themselves, some forms of treatment can be of a relatively invisible character while others are much more obvious. Williams' study and others such as Jobling's of psoriasis patients (Jobling 1988) indicate just how public some forms of treatment inevitably become. When they do, they often create new problems that have to be managed as part of the person's altered social situation.

The most obvious difficulty is when a patient has to have recourse to in-patient hospital treatment and thus to emerge from the often protective world of the home. Considerations of chronic illness and the hospital have, until recently, been a neglected area of medical sociology research. This has been due, in part, to the public health orientation of early work in the area, which has been counterposed to the growth of hospital medicine. While hospitals have been an important site for the exploration of social behaviour and the doctor–patient relationship in general, these studies have tended to be based in out-patient clinics or on life-threatening disease. Fewer studies in recent times have explored the dynamics of in-patient life (Album 1989), specifically with respect to chronic illness. However, some studies of chronic illness have begun to tackle the issue, including that of Williams on respiratory disease, cited above (S. Williams 1993), and these show how patients often approach hospitals with the same mixture of relief and apprehension that initial clinic contacts may involve. Relief may be evident because people are often admitted to hospital at a time when they are most ill and therefore welcome the chance of respite, further treatment and the alleviation of symptoms. On the other hand, hospitals constitute circumstances in which patients may become apprehensive, especially when treatment fails to help adaptation.

Strauss and Corbin, in reviewing these dilemmas, have pointed to the problems of hospital organisation and its relationship with chronic illness (Strauss and Corbin 1988). These writers argue that the hospital has traditionally been organised around a model of acute illness which is inappropriate in a period of rapid change, both in morbidity patterns and in social expectations. The boundaries between acute and chronic illness are now more faint than they were, as the example of leukaemia cited above indicated and as work on other conditions, such as chronic renal failure, has shown (J. Morgan 1988). As hospitals face an increasing proportion of their workload comprising chronic illness and as effective treatments expand (Gerhardt 1990), their organisation and culture will need to become more conducive to patients' needs. The importance of contextual and biographical features of chronic illness suggests that the traditional boundaries between the internal worlds of the hospital and the external world of the patient will also become weaker. The role of the family and others connected with the patient will have to be taken into account within the framework of the hospital itself. Developments such as specialist clinical nursing posts, which link the hospital, community-based nursing and the patient, illustrate the organisational changes that are now under way as hospitals attempt to relate more closely to the long-term nature of patient management and adaptation in chronic illness.

Coping, strategy and style in adaptation

Whatever the level of medical involvement in the long-term management of chronic illness and disability, the goal of most individuals is actively to achieve the best quality of life possible, in adapting to the condition. While the socio-medical model was largely preoccupied in documenting population level needs in order to identify resource requirements, medical sociologists have been concerned to document the active steps people take to achieve a level of normal life. This has not only been to inform the goals of service development, but also to point up the links between illness, disability and the wider culture. An emphasis on 'problems' has therefore been matched by what Corbin and Strauss have called the process of 'comeback' within a negotiation model of social behaviour (Corbin and Strauss 1991). As argued earlier, while medical care may be important to people at various points in this process, as Gerhardt has pointed out, in sociological analysis 'the patient's management of their illness is deemed, in principle, independent from what the doctor does for them' (Gerhardt 1989: 150).

In using the term 'comeback' Corbin and Strauss have drawn attention to the physical and biographical processes in achieving a satisfactory life in the face of illness and disability. By 'physical' they mean in this context the active 'work' involved in undertaking medical treatment and rehabilitation, often public in character. By 'biographical' they mean the attempts to 'reknit the past with the present and the future' (Corbin and Strauss 1991: 142) which have a more private and subjective character. For the present purposes, these two central aspects of 'comeback' may be seen to underpin dimensions of adaptation that bridge self, identity and social action. Adaptation rather than the adoption of a 'deviant identity' is emphasised within the negotiation model, pointing up the 'challenge to lifestyle and identity' involved in such illnesses and the active responses people make in order to manage them (Gerhardt 1989:139). These responses have been summarised in terms of *coping*, *strategy* and *style* (Bury 1991).

Coping

The term 'coping' has been widely used in the medical and psychological literature to cover a range of adaptive behaviours and strategies. One of the main problems with the use of this term has been its *normative* character, with its associations of 'successful' and 'unsuccessful' responses to chronic illness and disability. In everyday settings, both lay and professional, the idea of someone 'coping well' or being a 'coper' can often still be heard. As has been argued elsewhere in this book, the moral framework in which health is experienced makes such everyday judgements almost inevitable. However, as Radley (1994) has noted, this 'dispositional approach', focusing on the personality of the individual, has largely been abandoned in many forms of professional discourse, especially in psychology (Radley 1994: 148). This reflects a more relativistic moral climate, which emphasises different kinds of adaptation rather than success or failure. Following this and the work of Lazarus (1985), Radley goes on to distinguish 'problem-based coping' and 'emotional-based coping' (ibid.). The former refers to the strategies people adopt, which are discussed below, while the latter refers to the ways in which people maintain or recover a sense of self-worth. It is to this aspect of adaptation to chronic illness that coping most appropriately refers, emphasising the ways people 'put up' with illness and disability in the comeback process.

Restricting the term 'coping' to this level of adaptation brings into focus cognitive as well as emotional mechanisms. Drawing on Antonovsky's idea of a 'sense of coherence', Totman (1990) has summarised these as producing a feeling of confidence that the 'internal and external environments are predictable' (Totman 1990: 151). It requires considerable effort to come to terms with the limitations involved in changes to the body and social relationships (Corbin and Strauss 1991: 142). Corbin and Strauss also point to the components of identity, 'reconstruction' and 'biographical recasting', in efforts to bring the past, present and future into a satisfactory balance (ibid.).

A number of factors have been found to affect these processes in empirical studies, including, of course, the nature of the disorder or disability itself. Scambler and Hopkins (1988) for example, in a study of epilepsy, have shown how the nature of seizures influences self-identity. Not surprisingly, when they are frequent their impact is likely to be greater than when they are not. In the latter case the disorder can be more easily disguised and 'normalised', in the sense of assimilating it relatively easily into the person's existing circumstances, though there may come a point where the question as to whether the person still suffers from epilepsy or not becomes problematic. Kelly (1992), in his study of colitis, has made the point that in addition to the severity of symptoms and their potentially stigmatising effects, coping also involves a complex mixture of value orientation and outlook, with some patients 'coming to terms' more easily than others. As in studies of other conditions such as diabetes (Kelleher 1988), Kelly notes the tendency among some to incorporate the illness into an altered sense of self and in others to resistance, where the illness is held at a distance from the self.

Strategies

Coping mechanisms are bound to spill over into the strategies that people adopt in order to manage the problems their condition entails. Those who do eventually 'come to terms' will attempt to mobilise resources more openly than those who do not. However, it is important in mapping such responses not to repeat the normative tone of earlier approaches to 'coping'. In fact, no simple judgement can be made when the social contexts for action vary. Withdrawal from social activities may be as rational a defence against stigma and disadvantageous circumstances as active engagement. The image of the active 'go-getting' person, living 'successfully' with chronic illness or disability (especially those in celebrity or media circles) may only serve to reinforce negative reactions, both by self and others, where 'failure' to adapt occurs. Adopting positive strategies may be particularly attractive where previous 'life satisfaction' has been high and where current material circumstances are favourable.

In fact, the term 'strategy' brings the 'rules and resources' of social hierarchies more clearly into focus than the term 'coping'. Whilst 'resources' can refer to the energy and effort individuals expend in adapting, it also directs attention to the level of support available from the wider social environment. In Williams' study of chronic respiratory disorder (COAD) for example, while people (many of them elderly) spoke of their efforts in 'pacing' and 'chopping up' tasks to make them manageable and of the difficulties in balancing this with the desire to 'keep up' (S. Williams 1993: 27), the role of material factors and social support and social networks were seen to be critical to the outcome. It will come as little surprise that those experiencing most 'handicap' from their condition were those in the poorest circumstance (Williams and Bury 1989: 116). The interaction between social disadvantage, the onset of respiratory disorder and the additional material burden it creates, discussed at the beginning of this chapter, was here underlined in a study of London inhabitants in the late 1980s.

Moreover, few of the 92 respondents in Williams' study reported any help from social networks in managing the illness, even when, in pre illness settings, these had been in existence (S. Williams 1993: 18). Only a quarter of respondents who still had such a network were receiving support from it at the time of interview. As in much other work on social support and illness, it was the spouse who provided the vast bulk of the day-to-day help. Loss of wider social contact was also shown to be characteristic of experience in this study, with respondents poignantly describing who their 'real friends were' in times of trouble. M. Morgan (1989) has also shown that with time the emotional support needed at the outset of an illness is replaced by attempts to mobilise a looser set of social contacts.

Style

The question of resources relates closely to the development of different 'styles' of managing chronic illness. The 'performance' that is required of people living with illness and disability involves planning, rehearsal and evaluation of actions, undertaken 'with other people in mind' (Corbin and Strauss 1991: 144). In this sense, the long-standing sociological interest – from Mead to Goffman and beyond – in identity as the product of action and societal response is observed through examples where disruption means a 'refashioning of the self'. Here, again, such activity reminds us of the value-laden and moral framework which social behaviour in general, as well as adaptation to illness in particular, entails.

Actions are bound to be influenced by the level of confidence the person has in managing an altered situation, the expected responses by others and the availability of resources to tackle them. With substantial material resources and a supportive social network, forms of 'lifestyle' can be adopted which allow for a shift from an image of 'the disabled self' to one of 'the capable self' (Corbin and Strauss 1991: 151). Corbin and Strauss go on to list several aspects of 'discovering new pathways' in such adaptation. These involve 'a willingness to experiment with different ways of doing things', 'the ability to laugh at oneself' and the ability to 'pick up the pieces after a failure' (ibid.).

In a somewhat different vein, Radley summarises the same processes when he says that finding an appropriate style of living in the face of illness involves 'the need to resolve the competing demands of bodily symptoms, and those of society' (Radley 1994: 152). The interaction of two problems is at work here, namely the loss or retention of social participation and the relationship of self to illness. Attempts to adopt a style of self-presentation in illness or disability, in which the individual aims to 'overcome or defeat it', often requires, again, considerable performance in order to sustain an image of active involvement in mainstream social life (ibid.).

This may be easier in circumstances where symptoms are hidden and where the body is less exposed, for example at work among those young enough to be in employment (Kelly 1992). Other styles which involve accommodating to the condition and achieving some elements of secondary gain from the illness, as well as from withdrawing from social life, may be associated with those for whom their main source of fulfilment is outside of the world of work.

The possibility of adopting different styles in response to illness suggests an element of choice, despite the constraints that symptoms and social contexts may entail. At this point studies of chronic illness and disability connect with broader sociological concerns – with lifestyle, the body and health in a consumer culture – which have been discussed elsewhere in this book and are dealt with in detail in chapter 6. Within such a changing cultural climate, especially where the display of the body and pursuing health are important in claims to competence, new questions arise about lifestyles among those who may have earlier been barred from full social participation through illness or disability. These issues constitute a critical point where the ambiguities of change, as well as contexts for managing 'biographical disruption', are emerging. Developments in approaches to chronic illness and disability and in research are thus now taking place in a fast-changing setting.

DEVELOPMENTS AND PROSPECTS

There is now a propensity for at least some of those living with a chronic illness or disability to challenge their erstwhile 'deviant status'. As a result, there is a growing insistence on 'difference', reproducing and acting as a critical example of a more general process of relativising the boundaries between normality and abnormality, pathology and health. Demands for the right to participate in educational and occupational structures also suggest a collective dimension to disability which goes beyond the individual fashioning strategies and styles of adaptation. The growth of self-help groups, social movements concerned to advance the cause of the long-term sick and disabled, and media exposure all pay testament to an environment where disability is apparently no longer to be seen as a barrier to participation in the mainstream of life.

Current and possible future developments in medical sociology and chronic illness can be summarised under three headings. The first of these concerns the further exploration of 'biographical' and life-course dimensions, in the changing context of health and culture noted above. The second concerns challenges emanating from the disability movement in a more 'contestable' atmosphere that surrounds expert knowledge in this field, as in many others. Though such challenges have initially focused on the putative negative effects of medicine (and on specialties such as rehabilitation), socio-medical and sociological work have also come in for criticism. These challenges have aimed to expose the assumptions of research, especially concerning sources of social disadvantage. Finally, the implications of these changes for the relationship between researchers and the researched need to be addressed.

On the first of these points, work on biographical disruption, patient narratives and adaptation in illness has recently been extended to tackle key changes in patterns of illness as well as the cultural contexts in which they occur. Reporting on a study of 44 haemophiliac and gay men in Paris, Carricaburu and Pierret (1995) have provided new insights into the meaning and consequences of illness, and the resources available to adapt to it. HIV/AIDS has been regarded as, and indeed remains, a life-threatening disorder. Recent commentaries have pointed out, however, that in late modern societies initial responses to epidemics, characterised by panic, tend to wane as health care systems and policy makers strive to 'normalise' the situation. As a result, features of chronicity become evident (Berridge and Strong 1991).

In line with this, Carricaburu and Pierret characterise a-symptomatic HIV infection as a 'situation at risk of illness'; that is, having to live 'an apparently healthy life in conditions of uncertainty' (Carricaburu and Pierret 1995: 66). In doing so such individuals live out, in an extreme form, the tensions involved when the boundaries between health and illness become effaced. They explore, in particular, the 'biographical work' undertaken in order to construct a new sense of identity in the face of such stress. This is shown to involve (a) the management of 'the secret' of HIV infection, (b) the management of the constraints and restraints that the presence of potential illness involves in everyday interactions, and (c) the ability to find the necessary resources (both medical and social) in order to work positively on the first two aims. The authors also explore the timing and mode of infection: that is, the point of its onset in the life course and its relationship to the management of specific symptoms. The study shows that the distinction between 'felt stigma' (the fear of being stigmatised) and 'enacted stigma' (its actual experience) may be more complex than has been recognised. HIV positivity simultaneously involves the fear of the consequences and its immediate effects on social interaction.

In dealing with these problems, the respondents in this study variously mobilised what resources were available to them. The haemophiliac respondents had already adopted strategies, at work and at home, to minimise their existing illness, but in the face of HIV infection were being 'overwhelmed' and were withdrawing from social interaction. Gay men, on the other hand, were found to be more active, reaching out to friends and, where possible, relatives (Carricaburu and Pierret 1995: 78). Many of these respondents also had active and positive relationships with the health care system, though, interestingly, little direct involvement with gay organisations. Changes in diet together with the use of such resources as psychotherapy and spiritual support were also in evidence, as part of a changed and reconstructed lifestyle (ibid.).

Carricaburu and Pierret also show how some haemophiliac men experienced a form of 'biographical reinforcement', in reviewing their current HIV status in the light of previous chronic illness experience and future outlook. In this way they 'recomposed a sense of identity and tried to give continuity to their biographies' (Carricaburu and Pierret 1995: 85). Others, especially those who had achieved a level of 'normalcy' prior to HIV infection, now required a form of identity reconstruction in terms of the collective history of haemophilia. This often involved the fashioning of a 'victim' narrative to aid 'biographical reinforcement'. For gay men, on the other hand, the development of a more positive public discourse of 'gay identity' provided a framework for reworking their identities, 'as though homosexuals were integrated into society' (Carricaburu and Pierret 1995: 84). This marked a very different outlook for this group in comparison with the atmosphere of the 1970s.

Though there is not space here to do more than note the fact, interest in narratives and narrative analysis, mentioned here, is undergoing considerable development in mainstream sociology and anthropology, as well as in medical sociology (Riessman 1993; Kleinman 1988; *Social Science and Medicine* 1994). In medical sociology, for example, Kelly has recently examined what he calls the 'verbal accounting process' in the reworking of identity in living with chronic illness. Building on his research with patients who have undergone radical surgery for ulcerative colitis, mentioned above, Kelly shows that routines prior to treatment which helped maintain 'a veneer of normality' (Kelly 1995: 5) come under severe strain when contact with health services is established. Kelly shows that coping with these events and their aftermath involves ways of *talking*, in which people 'account for, explain and justify what they are doing and what they will do in the future' (Kelly 1995: 6). By collecting and examining a series of patients' stories, Kelly has provided an analysis of their narrative forms. These include appeals to an 'heroic status' in illness, tales of misfortune and 'disembodied' views of the self and experience. In each of these attempts are made to aid the presentation of self under conditions of uncertainty and moral hazard.

In this kind of work medical sociology has attempted to extend the theoretical and methodological frameworks that link illness and disability with self-identity, social interaction and critical features of the life course and social structure. The last includes examining the role of health and welfare systems, but it also refers to the impact of factors such as class and ethnicity (on ethnicity in chronic illness, see, for example, M. Morgan 1996). With the growth of medical and social research and its increased circulation in late modern cultures, however, gaps open up where new voices emerge.

The growth of self-help groups, campaigning organisations and social movements, not to mention the massive expansion of media attention and educational outlets, has created a new environment for the conduct of research on chronic illness and disability. The emergence of the disability movement, comprising a variety of political and educational activities, has been particularly important.

While at the political level campaigners have long used the findings of socio-medical and sociological research to argue the case for 'disability rights', more recent activists have challenged both the terms in which thinking about disability has been set, and the research process.

At the definitional level, the term 'disability' has come in for renewed scrutiny. It was noted earlier in this chapter that the term has long been regarded as problematic in that it refers to complex processes, overlapping with the related dimensions of impairment and handicap. Despite this, most campaigners and researchers to date have been able to put it to reasonably effective use. For some in the disability movement, however, the term now requires serious revision. Oliver, for example, states that 'disability as a category can only be understood within a framework which suggests that it is culturally produced and socially constructed' (Oliver 1990: 22). 'Disability' from this viewpoint is a function of those practices and perceptions linked to certain bodily or behavioural states that are so designated. Disability is not seen here as the result of chronic illness or trauma, but as the way these events are responded to and categorised by the surrounding society.

The important point for 'disability theorists' is that disability should be seen as a form of 'social oppression', not as an individual attribute or 'personal tragedy'. In a radical reformulation, 'disablement', Oliver argues, 'is nothing to do with the body. It is a consequence of social oppression' (Oliver 1996: 35). Relying on a mixture of Marxist labelling and social constructionist theories, the argument is advanced that capitalist society effects 'exclusionary practices' in relation to those activities and bodily capacities that are deemed unproductive. The problems of social competence discussed above are thus given a more critical interpretation. The tendency to portray disability as a feature of the individual, it is argued, reinforces an 'ideology of individualism'. Oliver states, in developing this approach, that capitalism has created a situation in which 'the construction of "able bodied" and "able minded" individuals' becomes significant (Oliver 1990: 45–46; Oliver 1996: 127). 'Medicalisation' processes are then added to this picture, providing a sharp attack on medicine's involvement in care and rehabilitation as nothing less than 'imperialistic' (Finklestein 1980).

While, as has been argued, some aspects of disability are clearly a function of social expectations and the impact of social structure, this is not always the case. It is difficult to imagine any modern industrial society (however organised) in which, for example, a severe loss of mobility or dexterity, or sensory impairments, would not be 'disabling' in the sense of restricting activity to some degree. The reduction of barriers to participation does not amount to abolishing disability as a whole. Only the construction of a thoroughgoing relativist position, in which 'difference' supersedes any notion of abnormality or pathology, can envisage such a situation (for a recent 'deconstruction' of deafness along these lines, for example, see Gregory and Hartley 1991). Moreover, the importance of chronic illness as a major cause of impairment and disability creates added difficulties in this respect. As Ruth Pinder has recently pointed out, Jacqueline du Pré's progressive inability to play the cello was not a function of social oppression or capitalism but the result of impairment, brought about by multiple sclerosis (Pinder 1995: 628).

From this viewpoint, arguments that disability should be seen as 'social oppression' present an oversocialised picture of the processes involved. Such an approach can easily gloss over social realities and reduce the complexities of individual and social responses to a unidimensional view of disability. In particular, it can systematically miss the point, made throughout this chapter, that the vast majority of disabled people suffer from chronic illness. Recent attempts by some disability theorists to recognise the importance of 'impairments' (e.g. French 1993, on variations in experience among the visually impaired, and Oliver more generally 1996: 35–36) suggest the continuing need for a framework for understanding disability that captures the multifaceted nature of changes in the body and self as they interact with wider social forces. From this viewpoint, the approach outlined earlier, which distinguished between impairments, disabilities and handicaps and the central role of chronic illness, would still seem to be of use in focusing on important aspects of experience. Recent exchanges between disability theorists and medical sociologists have gone some way in exploring the issues involved in making such links (Bury 1996a).

CONCLUDING COMMENTS

The implications of the above arguments for future medical sociology research are of note, and some concluding points can perhaps be made in this regard.

First, though medical research has been most frequently challenged by the disability movement for 'medicalising' experience, social research has also recently been portrayed in a negative light. Oliver has argued, for example, that 'almost all social research has been alienating' (Oliver 1992: 103). Although this comment is not accompanied by supporting evidence, its assumptions are clearly spelled out. Because those who are 'the object' of the research have not been involved in its execution, it is held, this adds to the sense of exclusion and 'oppression' felt by disabled people. The OPCS survey discussed earlier in this chapter (though developed in close co-operation with disability groups) has come in for particular criticism.

From one point of view this is surprising, as some disability groups have gone on to use the survey for secondary analysis as part of their own campaigning activities (e.g. Bruce *et al.* 1991, on the visually impaired). Indeed, it has been pointed out that campaigners such as Oliver have used the OPCS estimates (Bury 1996b). However, the activities (and research) of campaigning groups such as the Disability Income Group and the Disability Alliance in Britain have been criticised on the somewhat tenuous grounds that these groups are unrepresentative of disabled people in comparison with groups such as the British Council of Organisations of Disabled People (Shakespeare 1993: 260). Sociological work has also been criticised for not stating clearly enough which side it is on, and because it is still carried out by 'powerful experts'. As a result, interpretive research 'is just as alienating as positivistic research' (Oliver 1992: 106).

What seems to be involved here is the designation by disability theorists that all forms of research should be seen as a 'field of struggle'. As with other social movements, this may evoke the counter-charge that attempts are being made to displace one set of 'experts' with another (Bury 1996a). Indeed, the limits of the new approach to research may be evident, even to its supporters, where arguments 'gloss over difference in favour of the totalising and unifying role of oppression' (Shakespeare 1993: 255). It can also be argued that disability theorists are themselves arguing a case which reflects the experiences of a small and unrepresentative minority of the disabled. To repeat an earlier point, the vast majority of disabled people suffer from chronic illness, and this needs to feature as a central part of research endeavours. Moreover, the links between age, disability and gender need to be continually borne in mind (e.g. Arber and Ginn 1991).

Nevertheless, the challenges being made by some in the disability movement, in attempting to alter the research agenda and the relationships between researchers and the researched, are being felt in Britain and in other countries. As Shakespeare has further argued, the disability movement is articulating views – about autonomy, individual rights, consumerism and self-help – currently found among a variety of different social movements from civil rights campaigns to feminism (Shakespeare 1993: 250). In Britain much of the most recent debate has surrounded the Disability Discrimination Act (1995) which seeks to make acts of discrimination against disabled people illegal (see Barnes 1991; Campbell and Oliver 1996).

However, it is perhaps something of an irony that an apparently radical movement of this kind articulates values – especially those concerning individual 'empowerment' – that can be seen as central to the dominant ideology of late modern cultures. Having criticised approaches to disability for being individualistic, the disability movement finds itself championing individual rights and autonomy, without examining closely the moral and ideological ambiguities involved.

In any event, in the future it seems clear that (funded) research projects will need to take into account the political agendas of specific groups of the chronically sick and disabled more than they have in the past. The active involvement of 'client groups' in research design and conduct is rapidly growing. One benefit of the current debate is that the view that medical sociologists might have held earlier, that they were providing a voice for the voiceless, will need to be more carefully considered in the future.

This situation will also mean that the theoretical, methodological and professional commitments of medical sociologists will be scrutinised. The need for independent research on chronic illness and disability will need to be argued more cogently than it has been in the past. In particular, attachment to and the defence of methodological rigour will come to the fore, as it has in other areas of engagement with social movements, such as that surrounding the development of a 'feminist methodology' (Hammersley 1992; Bury 1996b). This chapter has tried to provide an overview of some of the approaches that have been adopted in the study of chronic illness and disability. However, cultural change and the growth of a 'contestable culture' suggest that research on chronic illness, as in other areas, is likely to remain a potential area for dispute as well as growth in the future.

Chapter 5

Death and dying

In the last chapter, the increased role of sociology in examining the demographic and health profiles of modern cultures and changes in medical practice, as well as in cultural change itself, were highlighted. The explosion of sociological writing on death and dying presents a comparable but somewhat different problem. Though death, as expressed in death rates at least, is less important today as a social indicator than it was in the past, sociological interest in the topic has grown considerably in recent years. Perhaps because of the fact that the extension of *physical survival* and biological death are no longer the overriding concern of the public health enterprise, death as a *social phenomenon* is brought into sharper focus (Mulkay 1993: 31–32). Whilst some of medical sociology's interest in the subject might be seen as a logical extension of work on illness and on professional–client relationships, broader sociological attention has reflected more general concerns. As epidemiology has moved away from mortality and death, sociology has moved in.

Of course, death is a constant source of threat and apprehension for human beings – 'the great extrinsic factor of human existence' (Giddens 1991: 162). It is also of interest to those who make their living from rehearsing, modifying and mediating such concerns. Libraries have been written on many aspects of the subject. But general sociological interest has until now been noticeable by its absence. While areas such as religion, education and crime have dominated the sociological agenda, death and dying have largely been ignored. The sociological preoccupation with social structure, meaning and action has emphasised the problems and conflicts of the present, and of the living. The apparently infinite character of meaning production and cultural renewal has rarely confronted its limits in death. Even the disruption of illness, as we have seen, is precisely what the term suggests: a disruption in meaning, not its end. The advent of HIV/AIDS, though it has reminded people of the dreadful effects of death in the young, has been discussed in terms that are wholly consistent with an active and combative view of life. As has also been shown in chapter 4, HIV/AIDS is now being approached as a chronic illness (the actual experience of death and dying in AIDS patients has, by contrast, received little attention). In this sense both mainstream sociology and medical sociology have seemingly shared the same view of being preoccupied with the problems of living. Death might properly be left to philosophers, clerics or even comic actors such as Woody Allen.

The rapid increase in sociological writing on death and dying, and in renewed medical sociology interest, signals a change in this outlook. Two interrelated processes may help to explain this. First, sociologists have, in recent years, been examining the processes and outcomes of modernity in ever greater detail. The legacy of rationality and the process of rationalisation in modern life have come in for particular scrutiny. The recent major structural transformations in modern society, including the fall of communism, the loss of influence of 'grand narratives' in liberal societies and the acceleration of globalising processes, have all challenged earlier assumptions about our conceptions of life and death (Lyotard 1984).

Most importantly, in assessments of modernity's legacy, German Nazism has continued to haunt both popular and academic debate, representing as it does the darkest moment in modern European civilisation, where death overshadowed life on a massive scale. In medical sociology, Gerhardt has explored the legacy of Nazism and the development of ideas about illness and deviance in the post-war period (Gerhardt 1989). She has shown how important Nazism was to discussions of normal and pathological social development as well as deviancy theory (Gerhardt 1989: 170). More general examinations of the holocaust, such as Bauman's *Modernity and the Holocaust* (Bauman 1989), have been supplemented by a wider examination of death and dying in late modern societies (Bauman 1994; Baudrillard 1993). Baudrillard, following Foucault, has linked rationality with the exclusion of 'death and the dead' in modern society; a process more radical, he contends, than that of excluding 'madmen, children or inferior races' (Baudrillard 1993: 126).

The second related issue concerns the millennium. As the twentieth century closes, the balance sheets are being drawn up. The tension between the promise of the century to usher in an era of freedom and (to use the much over-used term) an improved quality of life on the one hand, and the destructiveness it has actually witnessed (and not just through the holocaust) on the other, makes this a difficult task indeed. Generally, in many cultures, a 'fin de siècle' mood can be discerned, and this is expressed in an explosion of films, books and other media, portraying violence and death in ever increasing detail. These are often linked to a 'futuristic' vision of social conditions already observable in twentieth-century urban life. The development of destructive nationalism and racism only serves to underline the point. Despite being the last great taboo, death now seems to be *the* subject of postmodern writings, and postmodern society (Walter 1994). Sociological interest, therefore, once again appears to be following in the wake of societal recognition. In writing on death and dying at the end of the millennium, sociologists demonstrate an elective affinity with the growing and mixed sentiments of foreboding and hope for the future.

As will be shown, the value of this new writing and interest for medical sociology is double edged. On the one hand the increase in attention to cultural dimensions of death and dying provides a more fertile theoretical context in which to develop empirical work. On the other hand this may be misleading, as the mundane actions of lay people in communities (at least those that are relatively stable) and in the routine institutional settings within which death and dying take place may only dimly reflect the preoccupations of the wider culture and, indeed, of cultural theorists. Making connections between discursive sociological writings on death and dying and available empirical research evidence needs to be handled with care.

Against this backcloth, the chapter proceeds along the following lines. First, it examines in some detail the main historical/cultural approaches to death and dying that have emerged in recent years. In particular, it examines the influential thesis of the French historian Ariès on the rise of the private, silent and above all medically controlled death. Reactions to that thesis, especially that of Norbert Elias, will be noted. The importance of this debate to the development of critical perspectives on rationality and death will be shown.

Second, some of the main features of what has been called the *Good Death*, in contrast to the somewhat negative picture of modernity proffered by Ariès, will be considered. The limited evidence available on contemporary lay thinking concerning death and dying (especially about 'awareness') will be examined in this context. This will allow an examination of how far historical and theoretical concerns reflect experience and beliefs in 'naturally occurring' settings, and within particular contemporary segments of the cultural order.

Third, the chapter examines the question of awareness of dying in more detail, especially with respect to research in hospitals, where it has become a central issue. The tendency of many modern societies and health care systems (at least those of Northern Europe and North America) to adopt a policy of more *open awareness* about prognosis and death has received considerable attention, with respect to both the hospital environment and the wider community. The effects of changes and variations in hospital practice are discussed here.

The fourth and final section of the chapter looks forward to the themes and issues that are likely to dominate medical sociological research on death and dying in the future. Several important structural and cultural features of late modern societies, with respect to the care of the dying, are examined. The impact of hospice care, as an institutional expression of a more 'accepting' approach to pain relief and the dying process, will be discussed, together with changes in family structure and its influence on care. Specifically, the role that non-kin may (have to) play in the future is assessed, as families become more fragmented or unable to provide day-to-day support and care. At this point the chapter returns to the idea of the Good Death, and critically examines emerging views about personal autonomy and preferences, for example about the place (and even time) of death. These, the chapter argues, need to be set against the social constraints and dynamics within which such choices are likely to be made. It should perhaps be noted that though the chapter draws on a wide range of literature on death and dying there is not space to review the more narrowly focused and, to some extent, medically oriented so-called 'thanatology' research literature which has grown rapidly in the US in recent years.

THE HISTORY OF DEATH AND DYING

The discussion should begin, perhaps, with a definition of terms. 'Death and dying' may seem obvious enough, even stark, but they actually refer to a wide range of issues, many of them difficult and contentious. Some writers have argued, for example, that death itself cannot be conceptualised, as it refers to an unknowable and abso-

lute 'nothingness'. Death, from this viewpoint, represents the ultimate cessation of social existence, and therefore constitutes a major
threat to a sense of meaning in life (Berger and Luckmann 1967).
While we may be able to talk about 'death' in the abstract, our own
deaths remain fearful and finally impenetrable. For these reasons,
much of what concerns us in this area is dying and not death, the
manner of our death rather than death itself.

Yet, even though it may be almost impossible to contemplate or
talk of our own death, 'death' in other terms is intimately related to
dying. As has already been stated, the mode and manner of death,
including its timing and place in the life course, is bound to be
related to the dying process. Historical changes in disease patterns
have had important effects. Fatal infectious diseases, often associated with rapid death, have declined, and an increase in chronic and
degenerative diseases has brought about longer 'dying trajectories'.
Though much of the discussion here will be about dying rather than
responses to death (for example, mourning rituals, funerals and
bereavement) the two are inextricably linked.

In fact, recent writings on the history and 'cultural construction'
of death and dying have criticised the shift in public debate towards
playing down death and focusing on the dying process. For,
although the historical trend towards a more controlled, managed
and 'humane' form of death seems self-evidently preferable to a
rapid and brutal end to life, the expansion of professional expertise
and practice which has accompanied it has met with little enthusiasm. The exclusion and 'silencing' of death, particularly as the
result of 'medicalisation', has been seen as particularly problematic.
The work of the French historian, Phillippe Ariès, can act as an
exemplar of such an approach.

Ariès' influential book *The Hour of Our Death* presents a
panoramic view of death from early medieval times to the present.
The main line of argument in the book concerns a series of transformations in perceptions of death that have coincided with stages
of modernisation. Through an examination of various artefacts
that give expression to death in different historical periods,
including documents, paintings and literary materials, Ariès
outlines what he takes to be the main forms that death has taken in
Western culture. The culmination of this analysis is a wholesale
assault on contemporary attitudes and practices towards death and
dying. In particular, Ariès has been at the forefront of condemning
the superseding of death by dying, and the relegation of death to a

tabooed and professionalised arena. In important respects, Ariès'
ideas on death echo the more general tradition of critical social
thought discussed at the beginning of the chapter, in which modern
society and its associated rational view of life are found to have
failed.

Ariès demarcates five main forms of death in the rise of modern
society: 'tame death', 'death of the self', 'remote or imminent
death', 'death of the other' and 'invisible death'. For the sake of
brevity, a short résumé of each of these follows.

Tame death, which Ariès says dates from 'the earliest times',
refers to the most ancient approach to death. In this form, death is
'close and familiar' (Ariès 1981: 28). Being part of life and an ever-
present reality, death has to be faced and dealt with *publicly*. Here,
death appears in many forms, but is not, according to Ariès, 'a
personal drama but an ordeal for the community' (ibid.: 603). The
various forms this ordeal takes, in death-bed rites and burial for
example, allow death to be spoken about and openly recognised. It
is in this sense that it is 'tame'. Today, by contrast, death, though
apparently more controlled, 'has become wild' (ibid.: 28) in the
sense of being feared and unfamiliar.

With the development of modern society, a profound shift in
social organisation, religion and sentiment occurs in which,
according to Ariès, the development of individualism and the self
can be discerned. The *death of the self* refers to that aspect of this
new experience in which there is a change from an emphasis on
public ritual and ordeal to a more personal experience of death.
Ariès suggests that this change, dating from the late medieval period
onwards, means that 'the dying man attends his own drama as a
witness rather than as an actor' (ibid.: 109). Preoccupations with the
macabre during this period, and the emergence of such practices as
erecting monuments and tombstones and creating funeral liturgies
and wills, marked the emergence of an acute awareness, Ariès
argues, of 'physical death, suffering and decomposition' (ibid.: 138).
This has moved death 'by imperceptible stages from an awareness of
death and summation of *a life*, to death as an awareness and
desperate love of *this life*' (ibid.: 138–139, italics in the original). In
essence this means a 'shift of the sense of destiny toward the individual' (ibid.: 625).

Remote and imminent death refers to the development of the
above processes in the 'age of enlightenment', and thus through the
seventeenth and eighteenth centuries. Here, the growth of science

and rational thought is associated with the reduction of death in terms of 'magical and certainly irrational powers' (ibid.: 307). Humanistic and religious reformers 'dethrone and desanctify' death and it becomes, as with all other matters, 'subject to the law of moderation' (ibid.: 310), in which the rites of death are simplified. Ariès sees this period as the 'turning of the tide' in attitudes towards death, which despite (or perhaps because of) the new emphasis on 'melancholy simplicity' brings with it a sense of emptiness and fear of death. The separation of the spirit from the body, in turn, becomes associated with the rapid growth of medical practices on the dead, especially dissection. And the separation of death from life means that medical practice becomes increasingly associated with a perception of death as simultaneously remote and fearful.

During the early nineteenth century a romantic reaction to these changes occurred, in which the idea of a 'beautiful' death could be articulated. Here, the *death of the other* becomes a dominant motif, and is linked with love. Through a long exposition of such novels as *Wuthering Heights*, Ariès reveals the development of popular sentiments towards death; these, which in an earlier period 'would have been erotic, macabre, and diabolical become here passionate moral and funereal' (ibid.: 443). This change, according to Ariès, 'gave birth to a sensibility characterised by passions without limit or reason' (ibid.: 609). This amounted to nothing less than a 'revolution in feeling which seized the West and shook it to its foundation' (ibid.). Affectivity is now associated with *privacy* which gives a particular shape to the individualistic tendencies of the early modern period. These, in turn, are associated with a strong sense of the 'afterlife', and a form of 'reunion of those whom death has separated but who have never accepted this separation' (ibid.: 611).

Despite these major changes in feeling and outlook, Ariès maintains that in our own time the 'death of the other' has now given way to an *invisible death*. As the result of death being associated with love and intimacy, individuals have paradoxically lost much of the ability to 'possess' their own deaths (ibid.: 612). As the result of a belief in perfection, in which 'we tolerate none of the compromises of romantic society' (ibid.: 611), the 'solicitude of the family' and, most importantly, medicine take death over. As the result of an insufficient 'sense of solidarity', death has been transferred to the hospital, forcing it to become invisible and hidden.

In this final form of death, Ariès draws on Illich's (1975) attack on the medicalisation of death and the absence of community values. For Ariès, too, there is no real community today, for 'it has been replaced by an enormous mass of atomised individuals' (Ariès 1981: 613). Death has become sequestrated from everyday life, and dying has, instead, become the site for professional guidance and expertise. The main aim, for Ariès, is to try to ensure that this 'scandal' is exposed. Ariès' only note of doubt about this line of argument is found in his repetition of a question from Claudine Herzlich: 'Are people going to demand to die when they are ready to die?' (ibid.: 593). Ariès replies that 'we have no idea yet, but the very fact that the question is being raised is significant' (ibid.). However, Ariès' historical view of the changing perceptions and practices surrounding death leads him to suppose that any new approach is likely to extend individualism and confirm the absence of community and collective values. This view is shared by many sociologists now writing on death and dying.

There is clearly much to discuss in Ariès' views on death and dying, and especially his views of the loss of community. One way to begin might be to consider a counterpoint to them. This can be done with Norbert Elias' *The Loneliness of the Dying* (1985). In this book, written when Elias was over ninety years of age, a somewhat different historical perspective on modern society and its effects on death and dying is put forward, though many of the sentiments expressed are in line with the general thrust of Ariès' argument. Elias' intention is to show how his own more general theory of social development might be applied to death, and especially to the process of dying.

Elias' theory is expressed in another panoramic view of the development of modern society, from the Middle Ages to the rise of the modern nation state (Elias 1978, 1982). Elias' basic thesis is that the development of modern society depends on two interlinked processes: the pacification of society and the development of restraint over dangerous and emotional behaviour by individuals. The first of these processes involves, crucially, the centralisation of the means of violence in the hands of the nation state, and the second the increasing control and restraint in interpersonal conduct. Without these institutional and psychological structures, modern life, based as it is on an extension of interdependence among people and a complex division of labour, would be impossible. In earlier periods, people 'were less evenly restrained all round in the sphere of social life' (Elias 1985: 19). According to Elias, the subsequent 'screening off' of difficult areas of life, including death, occurred in a 'civilising process' unfolding over historical periods. Not only death but a wide range of emotionally laden behaviours became repressed in the process, especially those linked to the expression of strong feelings (including those of sexuality).

As far as death is concerned, Elias reiterates the point that 'death is a problem of the living. Dead people have no problems' (Elias 1985: 3). The 'screening off' of death from the living (including children) is not only part of the 'civilizing process' but is also underpinned by specific changes. Here, Elias refers particularly to the postponement of death to later life. Death for most young people and adults is now remote. The relative increase in security and personal safety, in comparison with the past, is associated with falling death rates and the increase in average life expectancy. As a result, death in old age and very old age has become the norm for the first time in human history. When this is combined with the tendency to increase the level of restraint over interpersonal behaviour, 'like other animal aspects, death, both as a process and as memory-image, is pushed more and more behind the scenes of social life' (Elias 1985: 12). Most importantly for Elias, this means that the dying are also 'pushed further behind the scenes, are isolated' (ibid.).

Elias follows many of the lines of argument developed by Ariès. The transition from a public to a private conception of death is the most obvious. Both Ariès and Elias see past societies as being at once more passionate and more accepting of death. The apparent unwillingness of people today to face the reality of death and the desire to render it invisible are also present in both accounts. So, too, is the argument that the transfer of death and dying to the isolated and isolating hospital room represents the final indignity of modern attitudes towards death. Elias' 'loneliness' and 'pushing behind the scenes' is close to Ariès' 'invisible death' with its emphasis on medicalisation, taboo and denial.

However, Elias identifies a number of problems with Ariès' approach, which he finds descriptive rather than analytic. Elias argues that Ariès' reading of the historical record is one-sided and, in many respects, caught up in a romantic view of death. According to Elias, 'Ariès looks mistrustfully on the bad present in the name of a better past' (Elias 1985: 12). The idea, for example, that people in the past 'died serenely and calmly' overlooks the fact that, for most people, alleviating the 'torment and pain' of death was rarely possible (ibid.: 13). In fact, Elias argues, the majority of the population would have died in dreadful agony. By the same token, while Elias also sees the change to dying in hospital as having serious unintended consequences, he rejects the idea that all medical care in this area represents a negative development. The idea of a painless death, he says, may not have 'advanced sufficiently to ensure a painless death for everyone', but it is great enough to allow peaceful death for many people (ibid.). Finally, while the 'screening off process' may hamper people's ability to deal with death and the dying person when they have to do so, the reduction of strong emotional involvement (for example in burials and the fearful exhortation of the Church) makes the balancing of gains against costs difficult (Elias 1985: 16).

As has been discussed elsewhere in this book, the ability to weigh up the value of medical developments and expansions in health care against their unintended consequences is indeed a difficult task, especially when changes over long periods of time are considered. But Elias' point is that historians who fail to appreciate social improvements when they have occurred may undermine their own stance. Behind such critiques lies a deeper issue, also identified in Elias' counter-argument, namely the difficulty in evaluating modernity and its cultural configurations as a whole. The putative negative effects of medicalisation and expanding professional discourse draw on and contribute to critical indictments of modernity. It is not surprising, to return to an earlier point, that writers such as Baudrillard and Bauman have recently written about death and dying in pursuing such an argument (Baudrillard 1993; Bauman 1992).

However, these views, as Elias argues with respect to Ariès, represent only one reading of modernity and of changing attitudes towards death and dying. Condemnations of 'mass society' and 'atomised individuals' sometimes smack of an elitism which has long been represented in some sociological writings on modernity. Attacks on rationality and medical science also run the risk of becoming contradictory, as ever more elegant and closely argued positions are proffered, appealing to the self-same intellectual faculties that they condemn (Bury 1986). There is in some of these writings a tendency to use historical perspectives to convey a set of romantic 'new age' and anti-scientific values that sit uneasily in a sociological framework aimed at an appreciation of contemporary realities and of their structural determinants. It might also be noted that critiques of modernity and its effects tend to be produced by people who have benefited greatly from modern society, namely those in relatively secure and supportive academic environments, which are a central part of its institutional framework.

While a critical appraisal of modern attitudes to death and dying is important, a recognition of alternative readings of the historical record is equally warranted. In fact, as indicated, Ariès himself seems ambivalent about the development of some of the newer approaches to dying and 'palliative care', against the backcloth of his historical treatise. His generalised approach to the present, seen as medicalised and 'tabooed', makes it difficult for him to assess recent cultural change and particularly the revival of public debates about death and dying (Mellor 1993; Seale 1995: 188). In citing the work of Kubler Ross (1970) – a leading psychoanalytic critic of the medicalisation of death – Ariès argues that this may act as a counter-weight to the 'exclusion' of death in modern societies (Ariès 1981: 592). At the same time he also suggests that such developments extend the remit of 'men [sic] of feeling and science, the new masters of the art of the dying' (ibid.).

Though new approaches to death and dying may well extend professional expertise and surveillance, Ariès provides little evidence about their effects. This is unfortunate, if only because of the enormous challenge to individuals and societies which managing death and dying continues to present. A more systematic and sociologically grounded appraisal of these developments is thus required. In order to pursue this, the idea of the Good Death, which has provided a way of focusing on some of the issues involved, can usefully be introduced at this point. Though, as will be seen, the Good Death relates to some aspects of Ariès' approach, especially to nineteenth-century attitudes, it is in marked contrast with his notion of 'invisible death' as *the* defining feature of modern experience. Difficult though the idea of the Good Death may be (it can understandably be read as a contradiction in terms) its use as an heuristic device can help to examine the experiential aspects of dying in late modern cultures. In this way we can move from a consideration of historical views to a more sociological and empirical approach.

THE GOOD DEATH

In Allan Kellehear's book *Dying of Cancer* (Kellehear 1990) and in an earlier article (Kellehear 1984) the author argues against the idea that death and dying in modern society are characterised by exclusion and taboo. The reduction of public rituals marks a change in social values and practices, to be sure, but this does not mean, Kellehear argues, that modern societies suffer from the 'denial of death'. It simply indicates that modern life deals with the universal realities of death in a different way from traditional societies. While individuals may deny death, or repress it in everyday life, no society can ignore death or deny its impact on the social fabric. Every society must organise ways of dealing with death and dying, and recent writings suggest, despite Ariès' critique, that no absolute trend towards exclusion can be discerned (Mellor 1993). It can also be noted that public attention to such matters as deaths from AIDS (Small 1993), the national grieving over disasters such as Hillsborough in Britain (Walter 1991) and the international reaction to the ferry disaster in the Baltic in 1994 suggest that the public discourse on death is not characterised by silence and taboo. Moreover, the tendency of late modern societies to try to reduce the amount of suffering and grief for individuals in the face of death, and to develop greater sensitivity towards the dying process, need not be dismissed outright, as Ariès does, merely as a form of collective 'pathology'.

The idea of the Good Death expresses the strain towards a greater sense of openness and personal control over the dying process, as well as the attempt to develop more humane forms of care. In *Dying of Cancer*, five features of the Good Death are outlined, distilled from the existing literature and, indeed, the longer European tradition of thinking about death and dying that Ariès describes. In particular, Kellehear has in mind an almost nineteenth-century image of the mixture of public and private forms of death, with family and friends at the bedside and with the clergyman in the background (Kellehear 1990: 3).

Kellehear's argument is that the image of the Good Death can act as an 'ideal type' against which descriptions of actual dying experiences may be set. At the least, it may help to examine lay views and the social contingencies that surround the dying process. The use of the term 'ideal type' should be seen as a methodological device, and not as a normative prescription about how death *should* occur. The chapter will return to the problem of values in this connection later. Kellehear's five features of the Good Death are as follows:

1 Awareness of dying. By this is meant both a personal and a social process of more openness towards the prognosis of illness,

where this is known to involve the high probability of death. Such awareness provides the foundations for other aspects of the Good Death and is important, according to Kellehear, if 'dying is to become a critical part of the dying person's identity and social relations'.

2 Personal preparations and social adjustments. This involves attempts to resolve matters such as family disputes, or arranging for someone to handle family affairs. Kellehear refers to this as the settling of 'emotional accounts'.

3 Public preparations, including finalising or checking wills, contacts with solicitors and, where appropriate, clergy. Here, Kellehear refers to the settling of more 'practical accounts'. This feature may involve the 'mediation or ritualistic duties' in which the individual puts practical affairs in order, for those that will survive.

4 The relinquishing, where appropriate, of formal work or employment responsibilities. Clearly the age of the person is important here, but Kellehear argues that sociological work on death and dying has neglected this topic. Although, as we have pointed out, most deaths in Western societies occur over the age of retirement, some forms of death (notably AIDS and some forms of cancer and heart disease) do not.

5 Finally, a Good Death involves making formal and informal farewells. These will be to both family and friends, and where people are involved in more formal care settings, to staff.

(adapted from Kellehear 1990: 47–55)

Kellehear recognises, of course, that individuals vary in their styles of living and social circumstances, and that these will influence the dying process. But these broad features, he maintains, are implicit in the literature on dying, and influence much of the developing professional activity now taking place. Kellehear goes on to examine these 'theoretical' aspects of the Good Death through interviews with 100 respondents dying from cancer. Overall, Kellehear finds that with respect to all of the main dimensions, and despite considerable variation in experience, 'such beliefs exist as ideals and as social pressures and expectations for the dying in their attempts to achieve the Good Death' (Kellehear 1990: 194). The Good Death helps to justify the actions of individuals, and acts as an ideology for professional practice (ibid.).

LAY BELIEFS ABOUT AWARENESS

Of all the aspects of dying mentioned above, it is problems associated with the question of 'awareness' that have received most attention. Of importance here is the nature of 'lay beliefs' about awareness that people bring with them to the dying process. While Kellehear's own study focused specifically on cancer patients, the assimilation of ideas about death and dying in the wider culture also requires analysis. The discussion which follows draws on a study of older people in Aberdeen carried out by Rory Williams (R. Williams 1990) providing valuable evidence on such beliefs in contemporary settings, which in turn may affect professional attitudes. This approach will also provide, therefore, the basis for moving on in the next section to examine the contentious issue of awareness of dying among hospital patients.

In his book on old age, Williams devotes considerable space to death and dying. Here, his discussion of attitudes towards death and dying reports on the results of his interviews with 70 respondents, set in the context of a larger quantitative survey of 619 people aged 60 and over (R. Williams 1990: chapter 5). Though some people in the study had experienced the death of close relatives, the interviews focused on beliefs about dying in general rather than the experience of death and bereavement, which was dealt with in a later chapter.

Williams' findings lend support to the use of the Good Death as an organising focus for understanding lay experience, though his discussion goes beyond the typology outlined by Kellehear. For example, though his respondents gave expression to the idea that 'self awareness with which death is faced' is an important issue, variations in response to awareness were found. Williams also emphasises that *control and timing of death* were important to his Aberdonian respondents. Williams notes that these two elements in lay views – awareness and control – stand in contrast to Ariès' views of the growing invisibility of death, and constitute a positive approach to the Good Death in a changing culture. However, he also notes that, in Scotland at least, these elements are also combined with a long-standing pattern of 'disregarded death' in which 'considerate deception of the dying' occurred, associated with transfer of control to medicine (R. Williams 1990: 120–121).

As a result of these tensions, Williams shows that a number of different values are held about the timing and mode of dying. First, people in the Aberdeen study expressed an *acceptance* of dying, in the sense that as the result of family traits or other factors people may have an 'allotted' time span. This was not so much an expression of fatalism but more a mechanism for facing the inevitability of death, as 'preparatory or consolatory' (R. Williams 1990: 96). Williams also shows how such acceptance among his respondents was held in a tension with the idea of controllability of death, that is, dying at the right time in old age, when preparations have been made. One respondent stated:

> he said he was going to prepare, have everything in order, and continue living. And he did so, and forgot about it; did all his preparations, forgot about it and went on living.
>
> (R. Williams 1990: 97)

As far as the dying process itself is concerned, Williams shows that Aberdonians held definite views of 'good and bad ways of dying'. These views could often be contradictory. 'To die the "proper way" was on the one hand to go quickly, easily, quietly, and unconsciously' (R. Williams 1990: 98–99) but on the other, the person 'should be cared for, looked after and among people, in light and warmth' (ibid.). In this way elements of the Good Death could be aspired to (public preparations, personal preparations and farewells), but at the same time expressed in ways that allowed the contingent nature of death to be recognised. Though sentiments were expressed that suggested that control over death should be exercised – even with respect to considering euthanasia – these were frequently contradicted by other statements, which gave strong support to the idea of not taking life (R. Williams 1990: 106).

In the crucial area of awareness and 'knowing the truth', Williams' evidence is equally multifaceted. His survey data provided the following replies to the question:

If you were going to die, do you think you would want to be told?

definitely not	17%
probably not	13%
might and might not	13%
probably	19%
certainly	38%

Together with responses in the qualitative interviewing, this suggested that 'there was a marginal preponderance of wishes to know, over wishes not to know' (R. Williams 1990: 108). In the above list, the largest single case was that of people 'certainly' wanting to know. But within a cultural milieu that still values 'disregard', 'the need for knowledge and the need not to say the awful thing' were not always reconcilable (R. Williams 1990: 109). Friends might feel that the needs of the dying were for silence, at the same time valuing the significance of last meetings and thus 'farewells'. As will be seen later in the chapter, the situation of friendship and dying may now be involving a variety of different experiences, under conditions of rapid social change.

In Williams' study, however, complexities abounded concerning what counted as knowing or not being told. In fact, in everyday settings such complexities cannot easily be captured by terms such as 'open awareness'. Williams states:

> Because of this complexity, one should not underestimate the extent to which a delicate resolution is achievable between the need to know bad news, and the need not to speak it.
>
> (R. Williams 1990: 113)

Williams summarises the themes and dilemmas encountered in discussing dying and the Good Death with his respondents in three main ways. First, there is a tension between a *natural death*, occurring when we are old and not too old, and a *prepared death*, when the right time has come and when we have prepared for it. Second, the Good Death could be in the form of either a *quick death*, where people die suddenly or without long periods of suffering, or *death after reunion*, where people close to individuals have spent time with them before death. Finally, there are the opposed forms of awareness, of *death aware*, in which people wish to know and are told, and *silence about death*, where the individual or significant others do not want to know or feel that the person should not be told (R. Williams 1990: 114–115).

In this important study, Williams gives some credence to Kellehear's idea of investigating the Good Death. In the context of Scottish experience, the nineteenth-century influences in this formulation, especially some of the more stoical elements, make particular sense, as many of the sentiments laid down in Protestant culture during that period still retain their force. Nevertheless, Williams notes that these beliefs were adhered to in a period of change, where developments such as the hospice movement (only beginning to appear in Aberdeen at the time of his study, though long established elsewhere) have formulated approaches which seek 'technical control without taking life; and . . . open communication without imposing it' (R. Williams 1990: 121). In particular, the question of awareness of dying takes on a greater significance as people adopt a less 'hidden' approach to death.

Against this backdrop of lay ideas and their complexity, the chapter now turns to the hospital context where the discussion of awareness has had a particularly sharp focus.

AWARENESS CONTEXTS AND THE HOSPITAL

The term 'awareness contexts' was first coined by the American sociologists Glaser and Strauss in their book *Awareness of Dying* (Glaser and Strauss 1965), reporting on a study of hospital life in California, although they had published a paper on the subject a year earlier (Glaser and Strauss 1964). Even though their work is now some thirty years old, it clearly anticipated much of the current discussion of the Good Death, including Williams' ideas of aware- ness and control. One of the reasons Glaser and Strauss took up the subject of dying was what they identified as the 'moral problem' in American society of increased knowledge among professionals (in their case doctors and nurses) and its transferral (or not) to patients. Whilst their aim was to address this question in a non- prescriptive manner, they state:

> Is it really proper, some people have asked, to deny a dying person the opportunity to make his peace, with his conscience and with his God, to settle his affairs and provide for the future of his family, and control his style of dying, much as he controlled his style of living?
>
> (Glaser and Strauss 1965: 6)

Part of the reason for growing disquiet was the fact that an increasing proportion of deaths were occurring in hospital. At the time when Glaser and Strauss were writing, some 53 per cent of people were dying in hospital in the US (ibid.). Similar patterns were emerging in Britain, with the same figure of 53 per cent of deaths occurring in hospital just five years later in 1969, rising to 64 per cent in 1987 (Scale and Cartwright 1994: 7). Fears of the 'medi- calisation of death' accompanied these trends. As was noted in relation to Ariès' and Elias' arguments, this was taken to mean a growing invisibility of the dying person, and a loss of social skills in dealing with painful experiences. Technology seemed to be taking over what had earlier been areas of human decision-making, to the point where death could occur only when the technological plug had been pulled, metaphorically and even literally (Illich 1975).

What made matters worse, according to these critics, was that the interpersonal aspects of hospital care were grossly inadequate in this area. Though people were dying in hospital, their professional carers had neither the necessary training nor the skills to handle the situation appropriately (Glaser and Strauss 1965: 4–5). Hospital medicine was too preoccupied with technical breakthroughs and therapeutic optimism to care about the dying. Such patients, it was held, symbolised clinical failure rather than success. Kubler Ross' controversial work started from similar premises (Kubler Ross 1970).

In its extreme form, the hospitalisation of death could be seen to constitute not only a set of general moral dilemmas but also a situation where specific abuses might occur. Sudnow (1967) for example, in a study of the routine practices surrounding death and dying in two American hospitals, distinguished between *biological death* and *social death*. The latter term referred to those practices that treated the person as if they were dead before the end of life had come. Sudnow alleged that, especially in the public hospital setting, dying patients could be abandoned in side rooms or even subject to the early stages of 'laying out' procedures before they had actually died (Sudnow 1967).

Whatever the generalisability of these findings might be, they keyed into disquiet about the role of the hospital in the care of the dying. Glaser and Strauss's approach to these questions was, however, less emotionally charged than much of the polemical writing at the time. In contrast, they set out to develop an understanding of the *interactional* difficulties surrounding the dying person and their organisational form in hospitals. Following writers such as Mead and Goffman, Glaser and Strauss were primarily interested in the ways social order could be maintained in the face of disruptive threat – that is, how orderly life in the hospital could cope with the 'unforeseen consequences' of the dying person. Here social order and rapid change were seen to be two sides of the same sociological coin, a theme in the study of health and illness which in different ways has been a thread throughout this book. For Glaser and Strauss, the study of dying in hospital represented one way in which 'the tendency to move out of regulated social bounds and into new interactional modes' could be examined (Glaser and Strauss 1965: 15). The conceptual framework of 'awareness contexts' provided them with a grounded way of approaching the issues involved.

In their book, Glaser and Strauss distinguish four main forms of 'awareness' which interaction takes in the hospital context. The first of these is *closed awareness* where, 'though the hospital personnel have the information' about the patient's impending death, the patient does not (Glaser and Strauss 1965: 29). The 'structural conditions' which underpin closed awareness contexts include a tendency of staff to believe that people do not wish to know that they are dying, of families to keep the knowledge secret and of information being systematically withheld from the patient. People who have no 'allies' in the hospital, either among staff or among other patients, are particularly likely to remain in a 'closed awareness context'.

Despite this, Glaser and Strauss make the point that closed contexts are 'inherently unstable' (Glaser and Strauss 1965: 38). The reason for this is that any change in the conditions that underpin them may lead to their demise. So, for example, new symptoms may contradict earlier explanations, or hints from the physician may indicate the true state of affairs (Glaser and Strauss 1965: 40). Though closed awareness helps to protect staff against having to deal with emotionally difficult situations, maintaining it past the point where it becomes untenable creates consequences of its own. For example, the patient may continue to talk of recovery and act accordingly, in a situation which the staff find interactionally uncomfortable. Such instability may be one reason for the emergence of the second and third forms of 'awareness context', namely *suspicion awareness* and *mutual pretence*.

In suspicion awareness contexts the patient 'suspects with varying degrees of certainty, that the hospital personnel believe him to be dying' (Glaser and Strauss 1965: 47). Where co-operation marked the earlier form of closed awareness, a tendency towards a more 'contested' situation now arises. One key area, Glaser and Strauss argue, is bound to be over medical information. Though medical personnel, and even relatives, may seek to 'shadow' the patient and thus reduce the chance of disclosure, patients were observed 'testing' staff by asking pertinent questions about their illness and its prognosis.

In time, a 'ritual drama of mutual pretence' is likely to arise, in which staff and patient both know that the patient is dying but pretend otherwise (Glaser and Strauss 1965: 64). This new form of awareness context again depends on 'structural characteristics' for its maintenance. Most notable here is a mutual avoidance of prolonged interaction and a consequent avoidance of talk. Physicians and nurses act in a way where they do not have to talk about death, 'and the patient does not press the issue, though he clearly does recognise his terminality' (Glaser and Strauss 1965: 67).

While mutual pretence offers a somewhat more 'serene' approach to dying than a suspicion awareness context, it too is an uncertain terrain on which to manage the process. *Open awareness*, on the other hand, refers, finally, to the situation in which the patient knows and indicates publicly that death will be the outcome, and staff know that the patient knows. Though this may be the 'preferred' mode of dying in the context of the Good Death and a way of countering the negative effects of hospitalisation and medical control, Glaser and Strauss recognise the ambiguities it brings in its wake. For example, though a patient may be openly aware of dying, the timing of death may be unknown or the subject of yet another area of closed or suspicion awareness (Glaser and Strauss 1965: 80). Second, the manner of dying may become a source of strain. For example, the patient may want to die 'pain free' or in private, while staff may have somewhat different views or priorities (ibid.). Differences in class and ethnic backgrounds may also influence the character of the negotiations in this situation. Once open awareness obtains, new negotiations between staff and patient may begin over the 'style of dying' (Glaser and Strauss 1965: 82).

What Glaser and Strauss go on to call the 'management of acceptable dying' therefore cuts across any simple prescription about its mode. Though they are critical of the consequences of closed awareness and especially mutual pretence, they also spell out the ambiguities of more open situations, especially the complex interactions and negotiations that take place in such contexts. This suggests that ideas associated with the Good Death, or 'natural death', are unlikely to be realised in any simple manner. As the earlier discussion of Williams' study indicated, lay ideas as much as professional ones have continued to express the ambiguity that characterises the need to know and the need not to speak about dying.

Glaser and Strauss's work on awareness has influenced a generation of researchers since it first appeared. One reason for this, as indicated, is that it deals with abiding concerns associated with dying in modern society. At the same time, much has changed in the period since their study of 1960s Californian hospitals. The most important of these changes in the care of the dying has been the influence of the hospice movement, which has been developing in Britain and the US for over thirty years. Indeed, one effect of this has been the development of a more 'palliative care' approach (based to some extent, at least, on open awareness) inside the hospital environment. Before developments outside of this arena are reviewed, the influence of this in studies of hospital organisation should be noted.

Field's more recent study, *Nursing the Dying*, (Field 1989) acts as a useful example, especially as it develops Glaser and Strauss's long-standing involvement with the world of nursing, as well as providing a bridge with wider developments in the community. The main concern of Field's book is the relationship between the communication of nurses with patients and the nature of ward organisation within which it occurs. While the disclosure of 'bad news' has largely been under the control of doctors, nurses are now centrally involved in the process and are likely to be more so in the future. Field argues that the growing trend towards open awareness in hospitals raises a series of questions, especially about *when* and *where* such news is given, and how its consequences are managed. Where Glaser and Strauss were talking about the predominant problems of closed awareness, Field examines the current emphasis on open awareness.

The shifting cultural background to dying is noted in Field's study, but the analysis proceeds, as did that of Glaser and Strauss, through an examination of the organisational frameworks of hospital and ward life and how they influence patterns of care. Though a section of the book is given over to community nurses, the central focus is on the hospital. Through observations and interviews on three hospital wards, Field examines the roles nursing recruitment, training and turnover and the organisation of work on the ward play in shaping communication with patients. Field argues that 'the care of the dying patients is directly influenced by methods of organising and allocating nursing work within hospitals' (Field 1989: 32).

Observed variations in the three wards studied lend support to these contentions. In the first, 'a typical surgical ward', its organisation had 'a strong adherence to routine' (Field 1989: 36). As a result, nurses' work was heavily routinised and the allocation of tasks fixed, making it difficult for nurses to get to know any of the 27 patients on the ward at any one time. A 'clear division of labour' was related to a principle of 'staff superiority' over patients, making communication problematic. Despite the more general trend towards openness, this ward operated in a largely closed awareness context which created difficulties, especially with cancer patients when suspicion awareness developed. Field reported communication between surgeons, senior nurse and junior staff as 'poor' and highlighted the particular problems this created for junior nurses confronted with dying patients.

In contrast, 'Ward 6', a general medical ward, was organised along 'team lines' with substantial delegated authority to trained staff. The Sister in charge of the ward operated with a more flexible or 'permissive' policy, where open disclosure of information to patients could occur (Field 1989: 148). Citing a study by McIntosh (1977) which found staff reluctant to adopt an open awareness policy, Field found that on this ward only 2 of the 16 qualified staff interviewed thought a closed awareness context was easier to manage.

Field shows, however, as did Glaser and Strauss, that emotional involvement of nurses with their dying patients, in an open awareness context, can be considerable. Moreover, communication with relatives was often made more difficult as a result. Field states: 'Whereas the nurses felt they could offer the dying patient something positive they often felt they could offer nothing to the relative' (Field 1989: 59). In terms of ward organisation, however, the process of care was encapsulated in the idea that the patient 'should not be left to die alone' (Field 1989: 60). Support for patients and mutual support among the nurses flowed from this principle.

Finally, the third ward studied by Field comprised a coronary care unit. On this ward a high nurse–patient ratio existed, as well as a more prestigious 'specialist' ambience. Related to these factors, ward organisation was again relatively 'open' with a high degree of individual nurse autonomy. Two patterns of death were characteristic of the unit: 'quick deaths', resulting from cardiac arrests, and 'slow deaths', resulting from chronic heart failure (Field 1989: 72). Rapport with, and support from doctors working on the unit were central to key decisions made on the ward, especially whether to discontinue treatment or not. As on the medical ward, most nurses preferred an open awareness approach to dying, but decisions about treatment in such situations were particularly difficult to manage with chronic patients. Field argues that the attempt to operate an open awareness policy once again involved considerable emotional involvement with patients and a flexible division of labour.

In summary, as Glaser and Strauss found, the structure of ward life, including its 'sentimental organisation' (Strauss *et al.* 1982), played a key role in shaping policies of disclosure and communication in Field's study. However, it seems clear that though both Glaser and Strauss and Field found that the majority of nurses expressed preferences to care for the dying in an open awareness context, it was more likely to exist in the later study than in the earlier. As a consequence, Field was able to show more fully both the 'unintended consequences' of this change in outlook and practice, especially with respect to communicating with relatives, and the benefits it could bring to staff dealing with an emotionally taxing and stressful situation.

Field's study underlines the point that the role of hospitals in the care of the dying is changing. The portrayal of the 'hospitalisation/medicalisation' of death as denying attempts to achieve a Good Death is, to this extent, becoming out of date. Rigid boundaries between the hospital and the outside world are less in evidence than they once were, with patients frequently moving to and from hospital care. Moreover, other work on awareness and hospital care has emphasised the growing attention to the emotional and psychological dimensions of the experience of dying in hospital (Perakyla 1989; Timmermans 1994). This contrasts with the somewhat 'rational' and organisational focus of hospital life in Glaser and Strauss's and to a lesser extent in Field's work.

Having said this, for many people hospital care is less central to the dying process than it was, with more now dying at home (Field and James 1993: 8). Within hospitals, hierarchical structures are also relatively relaxed compared with even the recent past, though doctors may still find it difficult to switch from 'the active management of disease' to a different pattern of care focusing on the individual (Field and James 1993: 12). Field and James argue that approaches to death and dying in hospitals have improved, though wide variations can still be found (ibid.). At the least, the traditional pattern of hospital care has been increasingly exposed to the growing influence of hospice and community care and changing attitudes towards death and dying more generally. It is to these issues that the chapter now turns in the final section.

DYING IN THE FUTURE

This chapter has shown how fears of the medicalisation of death and dying, as discussed elsewhere, have turned out to be only partially justified. Whatever the strengths of the arguments put forward by Ariès and others concerning the 'tabooed' nature of death and the exclusion of the dying, these have now been contradicted by developments which attempt to achieve at least some elements of the Good Death, especially more openness and greater personal control. In a recent discussion of the Good Death, Young and Cullen (1996) argue that: 'The authority of doctors to do what they like, and to maintain their power inviolate by keeping quiet about it [death] has been brought increasingly under question. The resulting openness has made possible a new kind of good death for more people' (Young and Cullen 1996:175). This is likely to be the pattern in the future, partly as the result of the social changes noted by Young and Cullen, and partly as the result of such developments as hospice care. At this point, the influence of hospice care and related community care needs to be considered and evaluated in a little more detail.

Hospice care, from the 1960s onwards in Britain and the US, set out to fashion an approach to dying in direct contrast to hospital care. Against the backdrop of impersonal care, routinisation and control by staff over emotional expression, hospices aimed to deliver 'more effective methods of pain control, an emphasis on palliative rather than curative care, and attention to psychosocial needs of patients and their families' (Seale 1989: 552). Central to this form of care was a greater willingness to operate within an open awareness context than prevailed in hospitals. Seale points out that pioneering work in hospices, such as that at St Christopher's in south London, developed a distinctive response to the inadequacies of existing care. It should be noted that a strong Christian ethos pervaded such developments and that for many non-believers, and indeed ethnic minorities with different faiths, such care was not an attractive prospect.

Seale argues, however, that its 'distinctive' approach may have been more apparent than real. A review of evidence from studies such as that of Hockey (1986) in the UK and Kane et al. (1985) in the US indicates, for example, that though attempts to follow pain control procedures have been made, practice variès widely. Similarly, with respect to psychosocial care, a distinctive staff approach could be found which increased patient control and autonomy, but variability meant that the general case for a developed alternative approach 'remains unproven' (Seale 1989: 556). As far as staff relationships are concerned, most of the available evidence suggests that, though a nurse-oriented and relatively non-hierarchical pattern exists in hospices, more work was required to establish whether such settings do anything more than hide status differences behind what one might call a 'palliative ideology'.

Such a picture of the results of hospice care may seem overly critical and rather 'grudging' in outlook. It is clear, despite the relative paucity of research evidence, that the hospice movement has come to symbolise, for many, the organisational expression of the Good Death. It has also delivered innovative and supportive services to many dying people. Yet not only does the research evidence suggest considerable variation in provision between hospices, but changes elsewhere are challenging the claim to distinctiveness.

In the first place, hospices have become the victim of their own success. When set up they have functioned on a local basis and appealed to a local sense of community for support, including financial support. With the passage of time, however, hospices have extended their remit from in-patient care towards setting up and encouraging home care teams, symptom control teams working in hospitals, bereavement services and, more recently, day care provision for the terminally ill (Seale 1989: 551). In doing so they have blurred the boundary between themselves and other forms of provision, running the risk of an erosion of their own identity. By the same token, as services have developed and as palliative care in hospitals has gained ground, so the hospices have faced increased 'professionalisation' and incorporation into health services bureaucracies. The success of hospices has also created a desire by physicians to develop a new specialty of 'palliative care medicine' which threatens, to some extent, to 're-medicalise' the process.

Mention has also been made above of the other side of the palliative care coin, namely changes in hospital care itself. The adoption of a palliative care philosophy and palliative care techniques is clearly emerging on a broad front. It will be remembered that two of the three wards studied by Field showed, in Seale's terms, that it is possible to have 'hospice-style care of the dying in a British general hospital' (Seale 1989: 552). It is difficult to say whether these changes have resulted from the direct influence of hospice care itself or from broader cultural changes towards more openness and 'informality' in a variety of different areas of life (Martin 1981; Featherstone 1991), linked to a reduction in the power of professionals. It might be argued that changes in hospital care would have occurred irrespective of the presence of hospices – perhaps as the result of consumerism and other processes influencing the Health Service and the doctor–patient relationship (see chapter 3).

In any event, many of the critiques of Western attitudes towards death and dying have failed to note or assess the character and extent of the rapid changes that have occurred and continue to occur in the care of the dying. Where hospice care was once a peripheral phenomenon, it is now part of a much wider set of changes embodying a marked shift in outlook towards dying. Some sociologists have regarded these changes, as with Ariès, as little more than an extension of more subtle forms of surveillance and professional control over the individual, imposing a 'new regime of truth' (Armstrong 1987). Others have reiterated the argument that such developments extend individualism to an unprecedented degree (Walter 1994). However, the simultaneous growth of professional care, struggles over resources and less deferential patients suggests that a complex pattern of palliative care will emerge in the future. In this context, attempts to achieve the Good Death will continue but will be affected by many factors, including continuing health care 'reforms' and the constraints of a growing managerial culture.

One of the main problems in assessing these changes is that much current sociological discussion has focused on either the organisational features of care or the social construction of death and dying. Little of the debate has been based on empirical evidence about everyday experience. It is one thing to appreciate the organisational aspects of dying in studies of hospitals and hospices or to speculate about the 'postmodern' approach to individualistic deaths, but quite another to explore first hand the experience of the dying, whether as patients or as 'lay' people. Indeed, the paucity of studies suggests that there may be limits, not only to achieving a Good Death but also to undertaking sociological enquiry about the sensitive processes involved.

One body of work that has achieved considerable success in tackling some of the problems through the use of survey methods is that of Ann Cartwright and colleagues (Cartwright et al. 1973; Seale and Cartwright 1994). These studies describe the last year of life of random samples of people who died in the years 1969 and 1987 respectively. Within the limits imposed by relying on carers' retro-spective recall of events, a clear picture of some aspects of change in experience has emerged.

First, the studies show that demographic and social structural change has had a considerable bearing on the experience of dying. The increase in longevity and changes in household structure between 1969 and 1987 have meant that spouses have increasingly experienced caring for people with chronic symptoms and with a reduced informal social network (Seale and Cartwright 1994: 219). Though official policy has continually emphasised home-based 'community care', the brunt of this falls on (largely female) carers. More of these respondents expressed a willingness to manage this situation in a more 'open' context, especially in the later study, but the idea of pursuing a general policy in this direction 'must be uncertain' (Seale and Cartwright 1994: 27).

Part of the reason for this is that, in comparison with the situa-tion in 1969, respondents in the 1987 study reported increased dissatisfaction with key areas of formal care that, theoretically, should have formed part of the official support system. Changes in the pattern of general practice care, for example, left people feeling let down, especially as home visits had declined between the two periods. Similarly, although domiciliary nursing was appreciated when it was available, those living alone and the very old (aged 85 and over) appeared to have considerable unmet needs. These poor experiences of formal care agencies cut across achieving a sense of a Good Death.

In the context of the present discussion, the experience of hospital and hospice care is of particular note in these studies. In the 1987 study only 4 per cent of the deaths in the sample occurred in hospices, compared with 64 per cent in hospitals. One of the most disturbing findings with respect to institutional care was that a sizeable minority spent the last year of their lives receiving few or no visitors. Seale and Cartwright comment that 'the loneliness of life before death in such situations compounds Elias' notion of the loneliness of the dying' (Seale and Cartwright 1994: 223). Such loneliness was associated with the more general 'travails of old age' and while hospice care may be part of a transformation of the care of the dying for some groups (especially those dying from cancer) it has yet to provide the basis for a fully developed approach to dying in very old age. Seale and Cartwright conclude their study by saying: 'The development of adequate services to meet the needs of this group provides an even greater challenge than that taken on by the hospice movement' (Seale and Cartwright 1994: 224).

Finally, it is important to underline the problems in managing death and dying which go beyond policy change and health care organisation, and which are inherently difficult for sociology to capture. While a rational approach to achieving a Good Death is clearly preferable to inhuman neglect or cruelty, it is clear from what has been said that such an idea cannot, in the end, be approached without a sense of ambiguity. Promoting the Good Death may do little more than disguise the actual experience of dying, as Seale and Cartwright show. The greatest danger lies in the fact that the Good Death, far from extending the remit of professional power, may act as an ideological gloss, covering the distress and agony that people continue to face with or without formal care. At this point, the theoretical arguments about death and dying, from whatever quarter, may appear increasingly abstract.

Prospective research with dying people, currently being undertaken in south and west England, is reinforcing this point (Young *et al.* 1994). In interviews with a series of 40 dying patients and 20 friends (who, in the absence of extended family and social networks, may take on greater significance in the future) it has been shown that many of the ideas of the Good Death have only limited applicability, despite their widespread currency. One of the problems encountered brings the discussion back to the question of definitions. In much of the literature (especially that on awareness) a presumption is made that doctors can determine, at a given point, that the person is 'dying', and then communicate this to the patient, who will then 'know'. However, the research at Royal Holloway suggests that such definite knowledge is often elusive and that the dying process is frequently characterised by uncertainty. In this study it has been found that some patients were admitted to a hospice only to find that after a short period of 'stabilisation' they were discharged home as 'no longer dying'. With changing disease patterns and developments in palliative care, the dying process becomes increasingly complex. Other problems abound.

For example, family members or close confiding friends may feel they are operating with a considerable degree of 'openness', with the patient involved in practical preparations and farewells. However, this may disguise considerable fluctuations in levels of awareness in the dying person. This is not only influenced by the uncertain conditions of the dying process, but also by the interactional and intense emotional difficulties which dying presents, even when it is clear that the end is near. Moreover, previous relationships may shape interactions with the dying person in powerful ways. Much will depend on such factors as previous degree of affection, level of trust, hidden tensions and even differences in status. For these reasons it has been found that at one moment the individual may openly discuss their own death and at another deny it, depending on the changing context in which accounts are required and who is being addressed (including those in interview settings). The relationship the individual has (and has had) with those around them appears to be as important as any of the features of the 'dying process' as such. In these circumstances, Rory Williams' depiction of lay ideas of the acceptance of death, yet not speaking its name, is reproduced in complex ways by the dying, especially in interacting with others. It also suggests that as sociological research attempts to get closer to experience, theoretical considerations fall away under the emergent and highly contingent nature of experience.

CONCLUDING COMMENT

The idea that new approaches to palliative care and better organisation of hospital and community provision can provide an answer to the problems of death and dying can only be accepted to a limited extent. To return to Berger and Luckmann's point, cited at the beginning of this chapter, death represents the most significant and finally unresolvable threat to personal and social life. Palliative care and sociological enquiry may both rightly emphasise the Good Death, involving 'empowerment', 'control' and the improved 'management' of dying, but emotional and social complexities are bound to remain intractable and resistant to all but partial resolution. As people (lay and professional alike) attempt to fashion viable responses to death and dying in late modern cultures, this intractability remains.

The desire for greater individual control, through forms of hospice-style care, devices such as 'living wills' and voluntary euthanasia, where people may attempt to exercise ultimate control over the place and timing of their own death, will, from this viewpoint, always be at risk of foundering. The last part of the present discussion has emphasised the acute uncertainty that characterises the dying process. The desire to exercise control, understandable though it may be, will always have to face the dilemmas which such uncertainties create. There is also a high degree of difficulty in balancing technical intervention and not taking life. Demands on professional carers to carry out individual requests to end life must be balanced against the collective sentiments of a secular society which place a strong emphasis on the medical contribution to preserving life. This is an important value orientation, even when the extreme and unpalatable forms of religious-based 'pro-life' sentiments are rejected.

The exercise of individual control must also be assessed in terms of its consequences for those who comprise the immediate social networks in which the dying person lives. For, in the final analysis, death and dying stand in opposition to life, including the complexities and meanings involved in existing social relationships. Fashioning policies towards the dying must always involve the awareness of uncertainty and the limits to individual control. Sociological research may be able to focus on these dilemmas but, like other forms of human enquiry, it cannot hope to resolve them.

Chapter 6

The body, health and risk

INTRODUCTION

In this final chapter an attempt is made to pull some of the threads of the book together by focusing on recent debates about the sociology of the body, especially as they apply to health and illness and related questions of risk. However, the status of 'the body' as a sociological concept is somewhat problematic, if only because the term is used in many different ways and in a variety of contexts. Although this book has attempted to map recent changes in social life, as reflected in the study of health and illness, it has done so largely through the recognisable categories of social structure, culture, interaction and the like. In each case, the shifting grounds on which the study of health and illness takes place – including the policy context – have been noted; however, it has also been argued that there are reasons not to abandon existing conceptual frameworks wholesale.

For example, while professional and scientific medical authority may not occupy the largely unchallenged position it once did in society, this does not mean that the power of bio-medicine has been entirely superseded by a more pluralistic approach to disease and illness, even though, as various chapters have shown, this is certainly in evidence today. While the distinction between health and illness may have become blurred, no longer existing in a 'strict binary relationship', to used Armstrong's phrase (1995: 400), this does not mean that *pathology* has become entirely irrelevant, either to medicine or to those suffering from disease. 'Health' is not, in any event a true binary opposite of 'illness', as it is more diffuse (subjective health, for example, may be good, bad or indifferent). And while concepts such as social class and inequalities may be more difficult to use in today's economic and political climate, this does not necessarily mean that society has entered an era of 'post scarcity values' beloved of some postmodernist writers. Indeed, the persistence of 'poverty in an affluent society' expresses many of the ambiguities with which social enquiry must now wrestle.

Having said this, a final discussion of the body and health provides a means of critically examining arguments put forward by those sociologists who *do* see discontinuity and fragmentation as overwhelmingly characteristic of contemporary social life and of sociological reflection upon it. Although it will be clear that the present author does not share all of their assumptions or accept the validity of all their analyses, many of the issues currently being identified are important and deserve serious attention. A consideration of the body, therefore, allows for an examination of some aspects of a changing agenda in medical sociology, as well as a changing society in the light of the discussions presented in previous chapters.[*]

Perhaps one of the most important starting points is to consider why 'the body' has become the focus of so much discussion in recent sociology. Though much is being written about the body, there are few accounts of why 'the body' appears to have become so important in social life. One explanation, according to Shilling (1993), is that, with the decline in 'faith in religious authorities and grand political narratives' and with the 'massive rise of the body in consumer culture as a bearer of symbolic value', a new 'reflexive awareness' of the body has become a central organising cultural motif (Shilling 1993: 3). In other words, as collectivist 'grand narratives' of modern social life and the schools of thought related to them collapse, so the direction of the analytic gaze turns inwards. 'Post-Thatcherite' individualism apparently reigns supreme (Samson 1995).

From this viewpoint, sociology is not so much creating an interest in the body as reflecting its growing importance in the wider culture, for example in fashion, the media, avant garde art, lifestyle and consumerism more generally. But even if this is accepted, it still leaves open the question of why sociology should pay the body more than passing attention, perhaps as little more than an epiphenomenon of cultural life. The importance of the body in the

---

[*] The author is grateful to the editors of *Medical Sociology News* for permission to draw on an earlier article on this topic (Bury 1995).

cultural sphere might be accepted, while still regarding it as peripheral to the main concerns of everyday experience. Various attempts
to challenge this view are now being made and form the basis of the
discussion which follows.

The influential work of Bryan Turner is a case in point. For
Turner (1984, 1992) the question of the body goes beyond sociological reflections on contemporary cultural trends. The lack of a
sociological account of the body touches on what he takes to be
fundamental concerns. He argues:

> The absence of the body from social theory is not an unimpor-
> tant or insignificant lacuna. The absent body implies and poses
> major problems for the formulation of a sociological perspective
> on the human agent, agency and human embodiment. If we
> adopt the idea of sociology as a scientific study of action, then
> we require a social theory of the body, because human agency
> and human interaction involve far more than mere knowledge-
> ability, intentionality and consciousness.
>
> (B. Turner 1992: 35)

Turner advocates a sociology of the body based on theoretical
linkages between the individual, self and society. He goes on to
locate this theoretical project in the work of Weber and Mead, and
what he takes to be their relevance to the consideration of fundamental human problems concerning 'suffering, joy, death, pain and
so forth' (B. Turner 1992: 36). Here the relevance of the body to
medical sociology begins to emerge, not simply as part of an analysis of the health correlates of lifestyle and consumer culture –
important though these are – but to the more deep-seated issues
that disease and illness pose for human beings. For Turner the question of identity is intimately linked with the body, and this is
reinforced by lay people's relationships with the technical sphere,
especially medicine. Developments such as those in surgery, especially transplantation, are of particular note. Transplantation raises
the issue of the person even having to contemplate being 'held
responsible for the actions of a body which is substantially not my
own' (B. Turner 1992: 37). It might be added that information and
preventive strategies based on the new genetics are also raising
important issues to do with the body, risk and identity. Lay people
may, in the future, be routinely confronted with evidence about their
biological inheritance and the risk of disease and about the bodies
of others, including their children and siblings.

The work of writers such as Turner, therefore, appears to be addressing matters of concern to medical sociology, revealing the interplay between 'discontinuities' brought about by social and technical development and the enduring concerns of birth, death and illness. However, while this theoretical focus in mainstream sociology on the body appears to be new, it may in reality be simply adding an extra dimension to existing concerns. Medical sociology, in particular, has long recognised the importance of biological and bodily change in illness experience, as has been discussed in previous chapters. The novelty of considering the body more explicitly in sociological analysis may therefore be more apparent than real. Moreover, while writers such as Turner have argued that the body has been absent in sociology, they have also noted that discussions of the body in other areas of human enquiry are not new, especially in some branches of philosophy and in social anthropology. This is an important point, as it suggests that mainstream sociology has failed seriously to consider ideas about the body that have derived from other important branches of human enquiry.

In order to contextualise the development of sociological thought on the body and its relevance for future work in medical sociology, therefore, a brief commentary on philosophical and anthropological approaches to the body follows. From there the chapter considers some of the main approaches to the body in contemporary sociology, and their potential value for some of the topics and themes of this book. The chapter finally considers the implications of a more clearly defined approach to the body for the future agenda of medical sociology. This centres particularly on questions of risk and the body and on sociological approaches to biological phenomena and the bio-medical sciences.

PHILOSOPHY AND ANTHROPOLOGY OF THE BODY

Philosophical perspectives

As far as philosophical writings are concerned, it is clear that the body has been central to many key arguments throughout the centuries. Descartes' writings are an obvious starting point, if only because they are so routinely criticised by sociologists for conferring on modern thought the legacy of a dualistic approach to mind and an 'anonymous' body, and implying an avoidance of areas of experience such as the emotions (Bendelow and Williams 1994). There is clearly an issue to be addressed here, as Descartes certainly believed that the mind (or the 'soul') was immortal and that damage to or even death of the body could have no real effect on it. Like Plato, Descartes believed *a priori* that 'the soul is by its very nature distinct from the body' (Cottingham 1986: 117).

However, the criticisms of the putative influence of 'Cartesian dualism', routinely reiterated by sociologists such as Turner (e.g. 1992: 37), fail to take into account the fact that 'the vast majority of scientists and probably most laymen too, would now regard Descartes' claim that the act of thinking or doubting "needs no place and depends on no material thing" (Shoemaker 1984) as simply preposterous' (Cottingham 1986: 119). At the least, a recognition of the interaction between mind and body is now commonplace, as the massive research literature and popular discourse on stress, for example, demonstrates. Indeed, Turner himself notes, in the introduction to *The Body and Society*, that few modern thinkers or scientists operate with a hard and fast dualistic perspective (B. Turner 1984).

The problem is, however, that anti-dualist views take many forms. For example, the philosopher Karl Popper spent much of the last period of his life working on the 'mind/brain' problem. In an interview published shortly before he died, Popper outlined a version of 'interactionist' theory, in which the mind could be seen to have a material effect. Basing his theory on Aristotle's theory of forces, Popper attacked mechanistic and especially computer models of the mind, arguing against their fundamental inadequacy. He states:

> We know that the mind is very closely related to the body, which belongs to physics, and that the mind therefore interacts with physics. . . . This we know, unless we are bad philosophers and try to philosophise these obvious facts away. In my theory, the question where physics begins and mind ends or where physics ends and mind begins, is most likely a pseudo problem. What is important is that they can interact.
>
> (Popper *et al.* 1993: 171)

Here 'anti-dualism' takes on an interactionist character rather than an 'holistic' one. This allows Popper still to see the body as 'physics', but without separating it off entirely from the influence of mind and treating it like a computer. However, this may not be the kind of anti-dualism that other critics of the Cartesian tradition have in mind. Indeed, one of the problems is that some elements of Descartes' own thinking can be regarded as a form of 'dualistic interactionism' (B. Turner 1992: 33). The weaknesses in such a perspective tend to be assumed rather than stated clearly. In addition, some medical sociologists have confusingly invoked an holistic perspective (Bendelow and Williams 1995) *and* an interactionist approach (Williams and Bendelow 1996), as if both are equally opposed to the 'Cartesian split' between mind and body.

Descartes was not alone among philosophers in being preoccupied with the mind and body. Others, especially in the nineteenth century, have also made the topic a central motif in their work. Bryan Turner, in his 1992 essays, notes the importance of Nietzsche's approach to the body for an understanding of theories of modernity, including those of Weber and Foucault. Indeed Nietzsche was somewhat preoccupied with the body, praising it in its healthy form and being obsessed with its ills. In *Thus Spoke Zarathustra*, for example, Nietzsche railed against 'despisers of the body' (he may have had Christian priests particularly in his sights) by saying:

> It is the sick and dying that despised the body and the earth and invented the things of heaven and the redeeming drops of blood. . . . Listen rather my brothers to the voice of the healthy body: this is a purer voice and a more honest one.
>
> (Nietzsche 1969: 60–61)

Unfortunately Nietzsche himself spent a great deal of his life concerned with the ailing body – especially his own digestive system – and its implications for our knowledge of the world. He also suffered from an ailing mind and spent the last eleven years of his life in a state of near paralysis in a mental asylum, dying in 1900.

It is noteworthy, in the context of health, that Nietzsche was not just obsessed with the workings of the body, but with diet, too. As Turner further points out, one of Nietzsche's aims was to contrast the way other philosophers 'stumbled towards the truth after enormous intellectual labour, [while] he danced his way joyously towards life' (B. Turner 1992: 2). Diet exemplified such an attitude. In *Ecce Homo*, Nietzsche wrote in 'humorous' vein that:

> The English diet, too . . . my own instinct is profoundly opposed; it seems to me to give the spirit heavy feet – the feet of

Englishwomen. . . . A couple more signposts from my morality.
A big meal is easier to digest than one too small. . . . One has to
know the size of one's stomach. . . . No eating between meals,
coffee makes me gloomy. Tea beneficial only in the
morning. . . . Sit as little as possible; credit no thought not born
in the open air and while moving about. . . . All prejudices come
from the intestines.

(Nietzsche 1979: 53–54)

Quite how far this is meant 'humorously' is a moot point. Of
importance to the present argument, however, is that Nietzsche was
trying to assert the importance of *experience* in everyday life against
the dictates of religious thought and of existing value systems.
Meals and walks were more important than grand systems of
morality. Knowledge and belief were, in this sense, less important
than action – at the least he suggested that ideas should be 'felt'.
Whilst it is true that 'action' came to take on more sinister meanings
with Nietzsche's notion of the heroic action of the *Übermensch*
('Superman'), his assertion of life, including physical experience,
against the dictates of pre-existing codes and values and against the
insignificance produced by the dictates of 'reason', was widely influential on modern 'romantic' thought (C. Taylor 1989: 445).

Equally important was the work of Schopenhauer, who immediately preceded and influenced Nietzsche (though regarded by
Nietzsche later as one who 'turns against life', Nietzsche 1979: 80).
Schopenhauer actually felt he had transcended the Kantian belief
that only the phenomenal world could be known, by rooting human
enquiry consistently in the body. The often repeated view that we
both *have* bodies and *are* bodies stems from Schopenhauer, and
meant that the *will*, with what he claimed were its disastrous consequences in producing suffering, can be overcome by attending to the
experience of the body – as the route to a fundamental underlying
reality (Magee 1987: 216).

As Zygmunt Bauman has recently pointed out, Schopenhauer
epitomises and prefigures the recognition and fear of the 'ground-
less' character of modernity, the will to power and knowledge and
the resulting absence of a fixed point for ethical life (in Nietzsche,
expressed later as the 'revaluation of all values'). If there is any
fixed point for such evaluation, Schopenhauer argues, the body is
perhaps the only one we have – for in our bodies we have a 'foundation' for addressing the world around us. Finally, and in line with

his more gloomy view, death (of the body) for Schopenhauer becomes 'the result, the résumé of life' and is 'a deliverance' from the world's lack of justification (Bauman 1994: 6).

In these necessarily brief examples it can be seen how philosophers have sought to link the experience of the body (and the mind) with knowledge and experience of the world. Although social theorists in the 1930s, such as Schutz, were influenced by the thought of philosophers such as Schopenhauer – the 'finiteness of the body' was important to Schutz in the understanding of meaning in life (B. Turner 1992: 85) – the body became marginalised in subsequent sociological thought. For those following the phenomenological perspective developed by Schutz, the body became a 'background' phenomenon, part of the 'taken for granted world' comprising everyday life (e.g. Berger and Luckmann 1967). While recovering philosophical thought on the subject is important in rethinking the relationship of the body with wider social experience, as noted above, it has historically had only an indirect and limited impact on the development of sociology. This may be partly due to the somewhat abstract character of much philosophical writing on the subject. However, as a number of writers on the body have recently noted, anthropology in contrast has offered a more consistent and contextualised approach to the body, and one which has had a closer affiliation with sociological concerns.

Anthropological perspectives

Anthropologists have had much to say about the body. Indeed, physical anthropology has spent a considerable part of its history classifying, measuring and even photographing human bodies, in 'exotic locations'. In the more recent social anthropology of writers such as Vic Turner (1974), rituals surrounding the body, often linked with key social transitions and 'rites of passage' such as birth, sexual maturation and death, have been documented and analysed. In this tradition, anthropological analysis has approached the sick body as part of symbolic repertoires concerning misfortune, alongside other 'natural events' such as disastrous weather, crop failure and so on, as well as being caught up in interpersonal conflict.

However, the body has also been discussed explicitly in a number of anthropological writings. A collection by Polhemus (1978) illustrates the range of anthropological interest in the topic, with essays covering body image, body adornment and body language, including gesture, dress and bodily 'expression'. Polhemus, in connecting the classical anthropological writings of Marcel Mauss with modern anthropological discussions such as those of Mary Douglas, states that it is 'Ill considered to argue in support of *either* a physiological *or* a psychological *or* a sociological approach', as there is 'a common ground of overlap between collective-social and individual-psychological levels of experience' (Polhemus 1978: 21). This argument for an 'integrated' view of the body, drawing on a range of materials, concepts and theories, reflected a common theme of the period, that of breaking down disciplinary barriers and developing more integrated approaches – including those addressing health and medicine (e.g. Eisenberg 1977; Engel 1977).

It is of interest to note that in pursuing an integrated approach, and in contrast to much writing on the subject, Polhemus offers some reflection on what is meant by the term 'the body'. In making a play for anthropology to lead a multidisciplinary approach, he wonders where the limits should be set. He asks: 'Can we really assume that the limits and boundaries of the human body itself are obvious?'. Rather disconcertingly he also goes on to ask: 'Does "the body" end with the skin or should we include hair, nails and other epidermal body products within the bounds of the subject? What of body waste material such as faeces, tears, sweat, urine, and hair and nail clippings?' (Polhemus 1978: 28). Mary Douglas (who has an elegant paper in this collection called 'Do dogs laugh?' dealing with the problematic distinctions between human and animal attributes) has elsewhere provided a detailed analysis of the symbolic processes of 'boundary maintenance' and the body, including those to do with 'waste and pollution' (Douglas 1966, 1973). However, the limits of what 'the body' is for sociology remains an important matter to which the chapter returns below.

In considering work in this anthropological tradition a detailed review provided by Scheper-Hughes and Lock should be mentioned at this point (Scheper-Hughes and Lock 1987). In their paper they develop a trio of concepts in order to organise and analyse the range of phenomena linked to the body. These are: the 'body-self', as it is experienced; the 'social body', where the body appears as a natural symbol; and the 'body politic' as part of social control practices. Their aim in developing these concepts is also to point to their relevance in the development of a specifically medical anthropology. Each of these concepts will be examined in turn.

As far as the *individual body* is concerned, Scheper-Hughes and Lock have in mind (as has been seen in the comments on the philosophy of the body) the idea of the body as the centre of 'lived experience'. Through the examination of anthropological accounts of the links between the mind, body and society, Scheper-Hughes and Lock point to the culturally variable and historically specific nature of the Western conception of the bounded 'individuated self' (Scheper-Hughes and Lock 1987: 14). Although Western societies often take for granted a strong sense of 'self consciousness of mind and body', other cultures and belief systems do not. For example, Scheper-Hughes and Lock point to debates about the nature of Japanese culture, in which it is held that 'the person is understood as acting within the context of a social relationship, never simply autonomously' (ibid.). This has further implications for the understanding of body imagery and the conception of parts of the body, both in everyday life and in the context of health and illness. Parts of the body ('particular organs, fluids or functions') may take on specific meanings within particular groups or cultures. Ots (1990) for example, in discussing Chinese health beliefs and practices, has spoken of 'the angry liver, the anxious heart and the melancholy spleen'. This approach to experience overlaps with the more 'symbolic' approach outlined below, though the boundary between the two is not entirely clear in Scheper-Hughes and Lock's account.

The *social body* in Scheper-Hughes and Lock's argument refers more explicitly to the symbolic meanings attached to the body, and especially to the way the body is used as a metaphor for social processes. This picture is gained from anthropological accounts in which – quoting the work of Manning and Fabrega (1973) – 'the confident uses of the body in speaking about the external world conveys a sense that humans are in control' (Scheper-Hughes and Lock 1987: 21). However, Scheper-Hughes and Lock contend that this sense of control has been lost in Western societies, where a dualistic perspective has been associated with a mechanical view of the body. Hence our tendency to speak in terms of the body being 'run down', 'wound up' or that 'our batteries need recharging' (Scheper-Hughes and Lock 1987: 23). Of equal note is the use of body and disease as metaphors in discussing the social and economic environment, in referring for example to the 'cancer of inflation'.

The *body politic* refers to the extension of the metaphorical uses of the body to the political realm. In this context the body is seen to be central to mechanisms of social control. Here Scheper-Hughes and Lock extend the work of Douglas to argue that when groups or societies are under strain or threat, the body takes on new meanings; 'the body politic is likened to the human body in which all that is "inside" is good and all that is "outside" is "evil" ' (Scheper-Hughes and Lock 1987: 24). More will be said about this later in relation to 'epidemic psychology' and the risk of HIV/AIDS. For Scheper-Hughes and Lock the current emphasis in Western cultures on the 'politically correct' healthy, young, thin and attractive body expresses the 'core cultural values of autonomy, toughness, competitiveness, youth and self control' (Scheper-Hughes and Lock 1987: 25). Health becomes an 'achieved' rather than an 'ascribed' status, with health disorders reflecting the failure of the individual to lead a healthy lifestyle. At this point it is possible to see the relevance of a growing emphasis on the 'reflexive awareness' of the body, mentioned at the beginning of this chapter.

The distinction between different conceptions of the body outlined here has become widely influential in anthropological writings. Byron J. Good's essays need to be returned to at this point, to provide a final and appropriate example of anthropological work on the body. Alongside Scheper-Hughes and Lock's argument, a brief comment on Good's approach to the body will point to issues that will be taken up in the subsequent discussion.

Opposing, once more, a mechanistic view of the body and of knowledge related to it, Good argues that the body, subjective experience and 'objective knowledge' are inextricably linked. He states:

Consciousness itself is inseparable from the conscious body. The diseased body is therefore not simply the object of cognition and knowledge, or representation in mental states and the works of medical science. It is at the same time a disordered agent of experience.

(Good 1994: 116)

On this basis Good argues, following Geertz, for the development of 'experience near' accounts of illness, which, he says, are lacking from the anthropological literature.

More important for the present purpose is that Good summarises the ways in which a coherent anthropological perspective on the body and illness can be developed. Specifically, he argues that the body should be regarded as a 'creative source of experience' in responding to threat, and that 'narrative, the imaginative linking of experiences and events into a meaningful story or plot, is one of the primary reciprocal processes of both personal and social efforts to counter this dissolution and to reconstitute the world' (Good 1994: 118).

Alongside this, as with Scheper-Hughes and Lock, the phenomenology of the body and its symbolisation also need to be distinguished and documented. Though Good is keen to retain a 'critical' perspective in analysing these processes, and therefore recognising the political and ideological aspects of the body, he argues that 'a great deal of the literature explicitly identified as "critical" is long on critique, long on program and short on real historical and ethnographic analysis' (Good 1994: 59). Again, we shall have reason to return to these comments.

To summarise this section, arguments by sociologists that there is an absence of the body in social thought, a persistent influence of Cartesian dualism and a need to bring the body back into social analysis are only partially warranted. Even a brief glimpse around the boundaries of the discipline of sociology has indicated a long-standing and, in the case of anthropology, growing preoccupation with the body. Not only that, but there are evidently clear links with at least some strands of sociological work, including concerns with 'mundane' everyday experience and with the symbolic uses of the body in social life and in mechanisms of social regulation.

For the moment, however, we may still accept, along with Bryan Turner and others, that despite all these writings sociology itself has not found a *central* place for the body as part of its theoretical apparatus, and that this has had an effect on medical sociology. In one sense this is true, and probably justified, though quite how far the effect has been negative is a moot point. After all, sociology's frame of reference developed precisely to draw attention to the nature of social institutions, social relations and culture that were *not* reducible to the individual mind or body.

It is perhaps reasonable to argue that the established disciplines of anthropology, psychology and biology were effectively doing enough on these latter subjects, even at the turn of the twentieth century. Much of the nature/nurture debate in this period occurred in the context of controversy surrounding eugenics, in which biological factors were seen, finally, in racial terms. In contrast, sociology was increasingly preoccupied with developing, in Nick Mouzelis' terms, a firmer understanding of *social hierarchies* in modern societies and the *rules and resources* that characterise them (Mouzelis 1991). Social structure and culture were portrayed as having effects on behaviour independent of biological processes.

It is also true to say that much medical sociology enquiry has concentrated on studies of hierarchies and resources. Debates, for example, on inequalities, the social relations of health care systems and the cultural shaping of experience in illness have reflected and contributed to mainstream preoccupations. Although, as argued in the introduction to this chapter, the body has featured in discussions of illness experience, this has largely been implicit. For example, though the nature of threat, particularly expressed in terms of mortality and morbidity, has implied the centrality of a physical dimension to social experience, this has not been clearly articulated as such. Much of the literature on social factors in disease occurrence and course (including work on stress), though bridging the gap between the body and the social environment, has not addressed this as an issue.

Having said this, it still needs to be demonstrated that a more explicit analysis of the body is of importance in sociology and in medical sociology. Those who appeal to the self-evident need to focus in more detail on 'the body' would help to advance their argument if they could not only define 'the body' more closely, as anthropologists have tried to do, but also explain why it should be paid more attention, given sociology's intellectual legacy. Even Turner, for all his advocacy of the body in sociological enquiry, suggests that it may be more relevant to concerns with 'human beings at a social rather than systems level' (B. Turner 1992: 35), though it is difficult to say exactly what is meant by this distinction. The philosophical and anthropological treatment of the topic alludes to a range of relevant issues, but this does not necessarily mean that sociology should establish different priorities in its analyses, or radically change its frames of reference.

In any event, calls to 'bring the body in' to sociological enquiry are now surely drowned out by the weight of sociological writings which are discussing the subject. Despite the problems in conceptualising the body, a large literature on the subject is now accumulating. The point is, however, that sociological interest is occurring in very different social circumstances from those depicted in the classical anthropological literature, as a variety of links are made between the body and key features of late modern or 'postmodern' societies. Whether these writings are constituting a consistent theoretical approach is a matter for debate, but their influence in some areas of sociology certainly appears to be growing. Before the implications of this for medical sociology are considered, the next section therefore examines some of these recent developments in more detail.

DEVELOPMENTS IN THE SOCIOLOGY OF THE BODY

Consumer society, constructionism and the body

Two main and related lines of argument have developed in discussing the sociology of the body in recent years, namely post-modernist and constructionist accounts. The first of these – postmodernism – emphasises the centrality of the body in consumer culture and in 'postmodern' societies more generally. While anthro-pology has emphasised common elements of the human condition and diversity in experience and expression, postmodernist sociology now locates 'the body' in a web of consumption, identity and self-presentation (in contrast to Schopenhauer) prised loose from any firm foundation.

This sets up a particular theoretical tension in the sociological literature, as writers discuss the importance of the body in the context of postmodern societies, while at the same time trying to use the body as a means of restating a 'grounded' theory of social action to include its biological dimensions. In arguments about postmodernism, however, the body becomes a crucial site on which and through which new and far less stable meanings are fashioned. Such arguments contend that the construction of meaning is occur-ring in circumstances which involve radical changes in social experience and social practice quite at odds with any notion of 'underlying' or 'invariant' realities.

To grasp the impact of the transformations that are held to be under way, Featherstone and Hepworth (1991), for example, have argued that three 'significant features' of postmodern cultures need to be appreciated in developing a sociology of the body.

First, they state, there is an emphasis in contemporary cultures on the cultivation of lifestyle or 'designer lives' in which 'consumer accoutrements', especially of the body, are constantly refashioned. Second, there is 'a playful and emotional exploratory approach to culture' involving a high level of consumption of signs, images and 'simulations'. And third, there is the emergence of a set of 'post scarcity' values in which the worlds of women, children, nature and 'otherness', once hidden, are what they call 'valid partners' on the social scene (Featherstone and Hepworth 1991: 375).

The example they use to illustrate these processes is ageing. Whereas, in the past, ageing and the ageing body were seen to be functions of a series of phases in a 'life cycle' closely linked to biological parameters – birth, maturation and old age – these are now seen as not being fixed, but part of a more fluid and negotiable 'life course'. Featherstone and Hepworth argue that 'Adult life . . . is a process we must emphasise . . . which need *not* involve a predetermined series of stages of growth' Featherstone and Hepworth 1991: 381). Although they argue, at the same time, that culture cannot 'mould nature in any form it chooses' (ibid.), the main point of their discussion is to show (as was seen earlier with Scheper-Hughes and Lock) that ideas linked with youthfulness and the youthful body are now pervasive.

This means that old age is not necessarily associated with a process of bodily and psychological decline. Age acts as no barrier to social participation, whether it be in fashion, leisure, sex or other elements of consumer culture. Chronological age is overtaken by how older people feel or look, 'from their own frame of reference'. Featherstone and Hepworth argue that the adage that 'you are as old as you feel' can now take on new meanings, as older people participate in the dominant youth culture and reject their marginalisation as the result of inevitable bodily decline.

Here, as elsewhere, rituals that have surrounded the body – for example those concerning age-related dress, fashion and body decoration – and have hitherto maintained the boundaries between social groups (including age groups) are being eroded and even inverted. Under the impact of global culture and especially the media, it is further argued, individuals can now shape their own bodies and lives, creating positive experiences where once they may have been designated as negative. A new 'vocabulary of motives' is emerging, according to Featherstone and Hepworth, 'which places an emphasis on the positive value of greater flexibility and openness, and a willingness to discard "chronological bonds" in favour of 'personal growth' (Featherstone and Hepworth 1991: 384). It might also be noted at this point that the elision of consumer culture and health promotion, among the elderly as well as among the young, brings health risk and body maintenance to the fore in these processes. Keeping fit and reducing risk need not be confined to the young.

Featherstone and Hepworth are aware that they are describing not so much an empirical reality, to be found in all segments of society, as powerful cultural trends. Moreover, their comments on the limits of cultural constructions suggest that they are mindful of the continuing power of chronological age and bodily decline, and its interaction with culture. As Bernice Martin has argued, even well-preserved 'summer wine' does not last for ever (B. Martin 1991). Nor do all those in a position to follow the path they lay out choose to do so, though resistance or opposition to cultural dictates of healthiness and youthful activity might be seen – like religion – merely as one further postmodern lifestyle option.

Reference to resistance and opposition brings forward the second and related line of argument. This is concerned not so much with the impact of global culture and the importance of 'the body' in consumerism, but more with the social construction of *bodies* in their various guises. If anthropologists have dealt with 'the human body' as a constant yet socially variable phenomenon, and some postmodernists have treated 'the body' as a key feature of late modern cultures, others arguing from a 'constructionist' viewpoint now wish to emphasise the construction of 'bodies' in the plural. Just as sex has turned into 'sexuality' and then to 'sexualities', so pluralism and fragmentation take another turn with analyses of the various discourses which fabricate 'bodies'. Here, theoretical consistency in sociological writings seems to be ruled out by definition. Grosz (1994), for example, argues that 'there is no body as such: there are only *bodies* – male or female, black, brown, white, large or small' (Grosz 1994: 19). Here, any idea of an underlying biological dimension in social life is regarded as nothing more than an ideological device, linking the power of dominant groups producing different forms of discursive knowledge – or forms of 'bio-power', to use a term taken from Foucault. As a result, there are now critical and largely separate literatures on the female body, the disabled body and the mortal body.

Take just two brief illustrative examples which bring the discussion closer to the themes of this book. The first, and perhaps more obvious, is that of feminist writings on the body. In contrast to writers such as Featherstone and Hepworth, who pay little attention to gender except in general terms, feminist writers have been arguing that key areas of women's experiences of their bodies have been powerfully influenced, indeed fabricated, through the ideological practices of institutions, particularly medicine, in a patriarchal society.

Control over women's bodies and their sexuality is seen in these arguments as central to the development of modern society, especially the splitting off of the private from the public sphere. Emily Martin argues, for example, that women are identified

> with the family where so many 'natural', 'bodily' (and therefore lower) functions occur, whereas men are intrinsically closely involved with the world of work where (at least for some) 'cultural', 'mental', and therefore higher functions occur.
>
> (E. Martin 1987: 17)

She goes on to argue that 'It is no accident that "natural" facts about women, in the form of claims about biology, are often used to justify social stratification based on gender' (ibid.).

In Martin's graphic account, based on fieldwork with women in the US, science and medicine create a series of metaphors, discourses and practices, particularly in relation to reproduction, that produce what she calls a 'destructive travesty' of parenthood (E. Martin 1987: 67). While younger women in her study were seen to identify with the medical model in areas such as the menopause, older women were more resistant, with some showing that they could 'even manage to harness the anger provoked by their position in society to their desire for a different kind of life' (E. Martin 1987: 177). The female body, for Martin, is a critical and indeed political issue. While postmodernists such as Featherstone and Hepworth would interpret 'resistance' and the fashioning of new lifestyles as part of a changing and potentially positive or 'playful' cultural site, signifying altered relationships between men and women, Martin has a more 'programmatic' view. She sees bodies in terms of the dominant discourses that sustain gender relations. For example, she argues that the language of contemporary immunology reveals that it is 'conceived in the terms of the era of flexible accumulation . . . and characterised by rapid flexible response'. Such a system of thought portrays the workings of the body through clearly demarcated male and female characteristics (E. Martin 1990: 121, 129).

The second example of constructionist accounts is taken from the field of disability. Here, arguments have emerged to challenge prevailing views of the disabled or 'abnormal' body and to locate the various discourses surrounding it, including, again, medical ones, within the development of modern society. As with gender, it should be noted that many mainstream sociologists have paid little or no attention to the implications of disability for their analyses of the body in late modern or postmodern cultures. To repeat an earlier point, 'the body' is all too often regarded as self-evident.

In contrast, Mike Oliver, for example, has argued that capitalist society has not simply been based on social class divisions (and, it might be added, gender and ethnicity) but on the construction of the 'able bodied' and the 'able minded' (Oliver 1990: 22). As discussed in chapter 4, Oliver suggests that this construction of the disabled body and person allows the system to exclude and segregate those who do not fit into its productive processes.

The 'exclusionary practices' that result from this are reinforced, for Oliver, by the idea that disability is regarded as a feature of the individual, as a 'personal tragedy' of a disabled body rather than as a function of the way society is organised. Medical knowledge, and especially rehabilitation medicine, are seen as forms of medical dominance which, with exceptions, need to be resisted (Oliver 1996: 106–107).

Not only this, but a number of writers on the disabled body have also sought to invert the categories that have dominated experience in the modern period. Just as 'black is beautiful' emerged in the 1960s, so a reversal of cultural attitudes towards disability is advocated in the 1990s. Joy Lenny, for example, has written that a psychology which suggests that disabled people experience loss with respect to their bodies does so from the point of view of the 'perfect bodied of body-image theory'. Instead, she suggests that there are 'increasing denials by disabled people themselves . . . who not only claim that "I'm in love with my body" but attack the medical intrusions that are part of all disabled people's lives' (Lenny 1993: 234). Like the work of Emily Martin, the challenge being mounted here is to dominant notions of the body as a product of discourse. It is also an invitation to invert prevailing perceptions and sentiments, bringing what was earlier hidden from view out into the open. This is in line with Featherstone and Hepworth's arguments, discussed above, that under postmodern conditions 'excluded' groups become 'valid' partners on the social scene. Paradoxically, however, this may mean that the body, far from becoming less important as a feature of social status, takes on new and perhaps almost obsessive significance as a result.

Preoccupation with 'bodies' in feminist, 'disability theorist' and other writing may evoke for some Christopher Lasch's charge of narcissism (Lasch 1979). The emphasis on subjective experience in the kind of writing reviewed above may reinforce individualism and difference rather than reduce them. However, the social significance of these arguments should not be overlooked. While they may often appear to represent only individual credos, falling foul of Byron Good's stricture that they are long on critique and programme and short on observation, their widespread and pervasive expression in more popular forms can be seen on a daily basis. The question that will now be addressed, therefore, is: What stance should medical sociology take in response to this burgeoning 'corporeal culture' and its expression in the various approaches now emerging in the sociology of the body?

MEDICAL SOCIOLOGY AND THE BODY

For some in medical sociology the answer to the question posed above is relatively clear cut, namely that 'programmatic' or 'constructionist' accounts should be developed, especially in line with Foucauldian precepts. This approach to medicine, as has been seen, is concerned with the ways medical specialists and other professional experts have developed powerful forms of 'constitutive' discourses of the body. Feminist medical sociology writings, especially those which trace the links between reproduction and power, are drawing on such Foucauldian ideas. Deborah Lupton, for example, following Emily Martin, suggests that a new agenda is emerging, challenging

> the notion that 'truth', 'knowledge' and the 'essential' female body can be perceived as universal. . . . Poststructuralist feminist scholars now claim that women's experiences of the body cannot be separated from the discourses and practices which constitute them, that there is no 'authentic' body waiting to be released from the bounds of medicine.
>
> (Lupton 1994: 160)

In this vision, no humanistic values can be pursued in medical sociology research because they inevitably disguise more or less subtle forms of (gendered) power. 'The body' does not really exist outside of the discourses (or medical 'gaze') that produce or 'fabricate' it. Moreover, all forms of medical care become suspect as they help to constitute the pervasive 'surveillance' apparatuses of late modern or postmodern societies. Thus public health, as much as clinical or laboratory medicine, has played a key role, it is argued, in 'disciplining bodies' in different periods of history (Armstrong 1993).

Through such approaches, the links between power, knowledge and the body can be illustrated, often using historical examples which 'deconstruct' a range of medical topics, exposing them to critical evaluation. The history of medical ideas about the body can be dealt with in this way, even though, as Christopher Lawrence has recently shown, the Foucauldian analysis of the clinical 'gaze' has tended to produce a rather limited view of medicine's involvement with the human body. Such an analysis has neglected the historical role of medical science and practice in political *reform*, as well as in surveillance and political conservatism (Lawrence 1995). We might also note that constructionist accounts also see little value in the scientific and organisational achievements of modernity. This, in turn, perpetuates the pessimistic philosophical thought that Foucault inherited from Schopenhauer and Nietzsche, in which the human will inevitably produces a restriction of freedom rather than its expansion.

While constructionist accounts are no doubt tempting pathways for some, they raise serious questions for medical sociology. In particular, the emphasis on discourse, and the resulting avoidance of the more mundane (but no less important) experiences to which they relate, may become a limitation (Bury 1986). In much writing on the sociology of the body, the erosion of categories or the inversion of meanings and a critical view of professional power have been developed at the expense of seeking evidence about the *experiential* dimensions of the body. As a result, the effects of biological processes and a balanced view of their medical manipulation in people's lives are missing. In short, and with few exceptions, much of the writing on the body has become frustratingly abstract and 'data free'.

Following the route of discursive analysis of the body and medicine, medical sociology may contribute new insights and materials, but it may also reproduce some of the more negative aspects of the sociology of knowledge that have developed in recent years. A preoccupation with the construction of knowledge may detract from its objects of enquiry, producing a sociology of science without nature (Murphy 1994). This has important implications for medical sociology. The divorce of analysis from detailed empirical checks on changes in bodily states in illness, or of the experience of medical interventions and their outcomes, may mean that a dialogue between the sociology of the body and medical sociology may produce a stance remote from social reality.

In contrast, this book has argued that medical sociology is in a good position to demonstrate the value of sound empirical evidence and grounded concepts. These can be gained from well-designed studies of the healthy and the ill, examining the relevance of the body in everyday life. In addition, *social variations* in bodily experiences need to be explored if connections are to be made with public debates about health, as well as related health policy issues. There is a danger of a large literature on the body developing that, paradoxically, seems to resonate with cultural trends but has little relevance outside of the strongly bounded circles of those committed to specific positions. This may turn out to be a move away from an engaged and theoretically driven sociology, to become part of a vaguely formulated approach to social life in which any kind of invariant or constant nature is strenuously denied in favour of a 'made up body' linked to a 'made up self'. Such notions overstate the more tempered arguments put forward by sociologists of late modernity that the body has become less 'natural' and part of a more 'reflexive' culture (Giddens 1991).

Recently, however, a more 'realist' approach to connecting the sociology of the body and medical sociology has begun to emerge. This is implicitly in line with some aspects of Byron Good's and Scheper-Hughes and Lock's approaches. These are drawing clearer conceptual links between the body, self, identity and the life worlds in which health and illness are experienced. Recent writings on chronic illness, pain and patienthood, and on the perception and evaluation of risk, whether from lifestyle choices or the wider environment, are benefiting from a clearer focus on some aspects of the sociology of the body. They offer the basis not only for illustrating some of the general propositions of the sociology of the body, but also for evaluating them. To round off this discussion, a brief illustration of these alternative approaches is given below.

Chronic illness and the body

Kelly and Field (1996) have advocated an approach to the study of chronic illness which focuses explicitly on the body. They argue that both social *and* biological facts need to be incorporated into sociological analysis of the body, and attempt to illustrate what is otherwise rhetorically acknowledged in more general sociological writings on the topic. They accept that although the body has not been explicitly excluded from consideration, it has also remained 'theoretically elusive'. This is the result, in their view, of an overemphasis on meaning at the expense of dealing with the 'restrictions and discomforts' of illness and disability (Kelly and Field 1996: 243).

In following this approach, Kelly and Field state that the body 'impinges on capacities in varying ways' and plays a significant part (alongside gender, ethnicity and other factors) in identity formation. The interaction between the body and identity alters, of course, over time, 'as human bodies grow, age and change' (Kelly and Field 1996: 246). Whatever the circumstances, they go on to argue, there is a constant 'corporeal' element in social life, in that 'to be acknowledged as competent social performers we have to be able to give the impression of some degree of control, use and presentation of our bodies' (ibid.). The importance of the biological dimension in social interaction involved here illustrates the continuing tension between 'ascribed' and 'achieved' status in modern societies (Benton 1991: 2). The making of the self is inevitably constrained by the 'ascribed' influences of bodily limitations.

The disruption occasioned by chronic or disabling illness, as was seen in chapter 4, throws these processes into sharp relief. As Kelly and Field argue, 'bodies change in chronic illness', and this means that 'coping with the physical body has to precede coping with relationships' (Kelly and Field 1996: 247). Reviewing a range of medical sociology literature on the subject, they show how people attempt to maintain a sense of continuity in the face of bodily change. Such studies show how closely interlinked a sense of self and the body are in illness – made more visible in such circumstances, but underlining their influences in social life more generally.

'Bodily contingencies' are, from this viewpoint, more than simply social constructions. Though the body may take on symbolic dimensions in human affairs and become caught up in surveillance mechanisms and social control practices, this is because the body exercises 'varying degrees of salience for self and other, through time and place' (Kelly and Field 1996: 249, citing Strauss 1975). In other words, the body would have little significance in social regulation if it did not have a deeper significance for human beings. Kelly and Field, emphasising the lived experience of the body, point to the extremes of the continuum of the processes revealed in chronic illness, from the case of someone with diabetes who can conceal self-management practices and thus assume the identity of a well person, to someone in a wheelchair, where 'their public identity is always constrained by the wheelchair' (Kelly and Field 1996: 249).

Thus the symbolic significance of illness arises from the varying ways in which it may or may not interfere with identity management. Of course, cultural stereotypes and stigmatising labels may, in turn, affect the ability to manage the contingencies involved. In Kelly and Field's analysis, the 'logic of the explanation runs from body to self to identity' (Kelly and Field 1996: 250) as physical symptoms do not always impinge on interaction; 'differently diseased bodies affect interaction differentially' as people may have to account for quite different bodily processes (ibid.).

Taking up Douglas' argument about the body and pollution, they note that people may have to deal with bodily matters (for example, changes in body image or dealing with body waste) that make *overlooking* or *repair* work in interaction difficult. They argue that under these conditions 'no amount of euphemism or politically correct discourse can detract from the centrality of the public and physical difference. It cannot be socially constructed out of existence' (Kelly and Field 1996: 251). While greater tolerance of difference may alter the salience of bodily (or indeed mental) variability within specific cultural segments, this does not mean that the body ceases to matter in social interaction. Far from it. As has been noted earlier in this chapter, the development of a more 'pluralistic' view of bodily 'difference' has at the same time been accompanied by a strong cultural emphasis on the fit, young and healthy body.

Risk and the body

The other theme in recent medical sociology that is relevant to this final part of the discussion concerns the links between risk and the body. There are a number of ways in which this is emerging in medical sociological research, but mention can be made of two examples at this point: risk, the body and lifestyle; and risk and the impact of medical treatment on the body.

As far as the first, risk and lifestyle, is concerned, this extends work on illness behaviour, health beliefs and health promotion. As chapter 1 discussed, the concept of 'lay epidemiology' directs attention to the way in which people apply their observations of the patterns of illness (in the example given, heart disease) to the physical characteristics of people thought to be at risk. It will be remembered that those interviewed in Davison's study of lay beliefs and knowledge identified a typical 'candidate' for heart disease in terms of their 'body type'; especially being overweight and red in the face (Davison *et al.* 1991). Thus bodily differences, as noted by Kelly and Field, have relevance for the study of popular perceptions of risk among the healthy as well as the ill, as people absorb and fashion information disseminated by health promotion experts. Backett and Davison (1995) have recently emphasised the need to see health-related lifestyle choices in the context of 'everyday cultural assumptions and processes which constitute social and physical ageing' (Backett and Davison 1995: 629).

As Burrows and Nettleton (1995) have pointed out, perceptions of risk of illness are linked with body maintenance, which in turn is linked with patterns of consumption, whether in terms of 'healthy' foods, alcohol, smoking or exercise. Lay people (especially in the middle classes) may combine a strong adherence to reducing health risks with high levels of 'indulgent' behaviour. As people become more aware and 'reflexive' about their bodies, they may emphasise aspects that are thought to be under their own control, while at the same time continuing to engage in high risk behaviours.

In part, this contradictory situation arises because of the inherent difficulties of making sense of expert advice about the impact of environmental pollution, contaminated food or 'risky' behaviour on the workings of the body. Much of the language of risk experts is couched in statistical terms, drawn from population level data. In everyday settings individuals often find it difficult, and anxiety-provoking, to try to apply such data to themselves and their families. The language of risk, based on statistical probabilities, rarely addresses the implications at a subjective or personal level (Kronenfeld and Glik 1991: 308; for a discussion of this and related issues in medical sociology, see Gabe 1995). Thus expertise itself becomes part of the problem, as lay people lose trust in expert systems to provide guidance through the minefield of information in a 'risk society' (Giddens 1991; Beck 1992). Linking 'lay knowledge' about risk with how people see its impact on the body may help to improve understanding of health-related choices made in everyday life.

Of all medical conditions that have become the focus of anxiety about risk and the body, HIV/AIDS is perhaps the most important to have emerged in the last fifteen years or so. There is not space here to review the now voluminous literature on HIV/AIDS, but when approached from the point of view of the body it exemplifies many of the issues discussed in this chapter. These range from individual changes in the body which threaten identity (Carricaburu and Pierret 1995) through the symbolic implications of the threat of 'pollution' from risky sexual behaviour as reflected in moral panics (Strong 1990b) to surveillance and control of the body in attempts to 'police' the condition (Watney 1987).

In a wide-ranging review of the sociological literature, Bloor (1995a) shows that, despite the difficulties discussed above, the level of lay knowledge of the risks of infection from HIV is consistently high. This is true even among younger 'men who have sex with other men' (Fitzpatrick *et al.* 1989). As with earlier comments on health promotion, one of the sociological issues this poses is the relationship between knowledge and action. It is clear that people make a range of calculations about the risk of HIV infection depending on the nature of their social relationships and on the behaviour involved in them, especially, of course, among those who are injecting drugs. This indicates that the links between the 'routes of transmission' of the infection in the body and 'unsafe sex' practices, or the sharing of needles, are generally well understood. However, some people (Bloor mentions evidence on bisexual men in this connection) may still underestimate the risks they are exposed to (or simply be willing to take them). There is also considerable cultural variability in risk perception. It is possible, therefore, that a clearer focus on the body, in relation to people's views of information available, might help in understanding some of the differences in responses to risk seen in the literature in the HIV area (Bloor 1995a: 60).

Bloor goes on to note the tendency of sociological studies of risk and HIV to concentrate on the 'linking of discourse and power', as part of a political critique of the 'policing of sexuality, the punishment of victims and the surveillance of deviants' (Bloor 1995a: 84). Bloor's own approach, in contrast, is to emphasise three other perspectives on risk: a social psychological model, in which 'health beliefs' are examined in relation to perceptions of vulnerability of the body to infection and generally to poor health; a sociological view of 'cost/benefit' assessment, in which the attractions as well as the dangers of risk are examined; and finally what Bloor terms, following Mary Douglas, a 'culture of risk approach, in which perceptions are seen as a function of learned orientations to risk found in different sub-cultures' (Bloor 1995a: 85). Bloor reviews these three areas of risk analysis and then adds a fourth of his own, based on a phenomenological/cognitive perspective derived from Schutz.

In this latter area, Bloor argues for a form of analysis in which the everyday world of 'hidden' routines and behaviours is put at the centre of sociological enquiry. In the case of HIV infection, he argues that the distinction between 'the social world of routine activities on the one hand and on the other hand the world of considered alternatives and calculative action' is particularly pertinent (Bloor 1995a: 97). This approach brings into focus, Bloor argues, the ways in which people facing health risks balance the habitual demands in situations which influence action (e.g. sexual, drug related) with perceptions or knowledge they may bring to them. The latter will involve, crucially, knowledge of the body. Moreover, such an approach can also be used to explain *changes* in behaviour and the ways in which 'recipes for action' have to be fashioned within the constraints that the individual faces (Bloor 1995a: 98, 99; for a further discussion and development of these perspectives, see Bloor 1995b).

As was seen earlier in this chapter, the approach to social life derived from Schutz's phenomenology has within it a distinctly 'corporeal' element, connected with the experiential and temporal aspects of the body as they affect the production of meaning in everyday life (B. Turner 1992: 85). However, as was also noted, other, largely cognitive, aspects of his sociology have subsequently overshadowed this concern with the body. In the case of HIV infection a clearer focus on the body would allow medical sociologists to address the *content* of health beliefs as well as action in more detail. In this way a 'social cognitive' approach to risk, of the sort advocated by Bloor, focusing on its 'embodied' character, could throw new light on how behavioural repertoires and constraints are learned and managed. Even though the risk of HIV infection and subsequent illness clearly involves the body in a number of important respects (e.g. sexual contact, physical and emotional intimacy, changes in the body with the onset of symptoms and disability caused by AIDS), these remain underplayed in sociological accounts. Their links with identity formation and maintenance, within the context of the behavioural 'trade offs' described by Bloor, could be made more visible.

Finally, in addressing the links between risk and the body, the question of the effects of medical treatments needs to be considered. Modern populations have to absorb not only an ever increasing amount of expert advice about their bodies and health, but also information about the treatments they may receive when ill.

The case of judging the risks and benefits of treatments also involves monitoring bodily changes and the perceptions that others may have of them.

Taking the case of tranquilliser use among people suffering from anxiety, Gabe and Bury (1996), for example, have distinguished three levels of risk. The first deals with the perception of risk in terms of the effects of the drug on the mind or body of the user. At this *experiential* level empirical studies demonstrate considerable ambivalence about the use of such drugs. Respondents in one study (Gabe and Thorogood 1986)

> stated that they were concerned about the danger of becoming dependent on or 'addicted' to tranquillisers and felt that they might be harming their body or mind by ingesting such 'unnatural' substances. Others said they felt these drugs were helpful in that they offered them 'peace of mind'.
>
> (Gabe and Bury 1996: 81)

As with Davison's study of risk and heart disease, people compared their own experience with that of others. In Gabe and Thorogood's study, people drew on observations of those they knew to be taking tranquillisers, as well as assimilating warnings about the side-effects of the drugs from the media and other sources.

The second level of risk identified by Gabe and Bury concerns the strategies people use in 'risk management'. People who are undergoing long-term treatment may be required to be self-directing (at least to some extent) in managing the regimen in question. Gabe and Bury argue that in the example of tranquilliser use patients tend to fall into two groups: those for whom the drug is regarded as a 'life line' and those who regard it only as a 'stand by' (Gabe and Bury 1996: 84). They also discuss Helman's (1981) anthropological approach to the question, in which he distinguishes between the use of such drugs as tonic, fuel or food. Risks to the body from tranquilliser use are managed through the employment of such metaphors in order to build them into the daily routines of the individual, 'tonic' referring to intermittent use, 'fuel' for use in crises, and 'food' for use on a regular basis taken at set times.

This kind of approach also relates to the third level of risk discussed by Gabe and Bury: what they call 'social risk'. This refers to the potentially negative risks people take in being seen as 'drug takers' and, therefore, as not being able to cope with everyday life. Just as in Kelly and Field's argument social competence may be questioned if the individual's display of control and presentation of the body is disrupted, this may also apply to the physical and psychological consequences involved in long-term medical treatment. The use of tranquillisers may be a 'hidden' dimension of the person's life (allowing them to remain outwardly healthy) but it is likely to be known about by family members, and over time by a wider network of friends. This may be regarded sympathetically, as confidants exchange ideas and information about the drugs, but it may also involve the risk of damaging the person's identity as a competent social actor. This level of risk suggests, as do the other two, that self, identity and the body may often be significantly affected by medical treatment, as well as by illness itself. Again, medical sociology can throw light on such processes in future work on illness experience and the body.

CONCLUDING COMMENTS

The argument put forward here, that medical sociology is well placed to examine how experiences of the body affect identity and social life, as well as how the reverse occurs, is likely to be treated sceptically by fully paid-up postmodernists and constructionists. As has been shown, the idea of an invariant nature, or underlying if changing biological dimension to life, is, for some, no longer a thinkable idea. Though writings on the sociology of the body often pay lip service to the role of biological factors, this is often combined with a form of theorising which presents an 'oversocialised' or 'overpoliticised' view of the processes at work. Much writing on the body simply avoids the incommensurate nature of perspectives being invoked. However, a 'realist' perspective which recognises the 'obduracy of the body' and its role in everyday life (Kelly and Field 1994) offers a clearer alternative to developing research in medical sociology.

Such an approach suggests the need for an emphasis on the constant and changing features of the human body as a physical entity, setting limits and providing capacities for people to act – that is, the body as the 'material vehicle of personhood', to use Rom Harré's phrase (Harré 1991: 3). This involves a definition of the body as the combination of physiological and mental processes and structures as well as 'surface appearances', interacting with cognitive processes and the social environment; a definition that can tackle head-on the strong relativism of many current approaches, which only see the body as discourse. Indeed, it may be possible in developing such an approach to move beyond an 'interactionist' view of the body and the social environment to conceptualise "'persons", who are necessarily organically embodied, but who also have psychological and social relational attributes' (Benton 1991: 5). Though this might suggests a return to the idea of an 'holistic' approach, the relationship between the different levels of experience can more properly be seen as constituting the realist view of the body being advocated here.

Without a proper account of what is meant by 'the body' and how the concept is being used, arguments which appeal to the self-evident realities of bodily experiences will not be able to inform empirical work. In much sociological writing on the body, its 'obdurate' and real influence on experience still remains 'elusive'. This chapter has tried to show, albeit briefly, the value of medical sociological studies in linking the body, risk and broader social processes. However, the connections between biological processes and the social patterning of health need not be confined to these topics alone. They provide a conceptual thread which can inform a number of the themes in this book, from studies of health beliefs to the questions of experiencing inequalities in health and lay people's responses to the doctor–patient relationship.

Finally, if medical sociology is to expand its traditional field of enquiry, to focus more explicitly on the body, there is also a need to rethink the relationship between sociology and the biological sciences as fields of human enquiry. The view that sociology all too often espouses, that biology – here the discipline rather than the underlying entities or realities to which it refers – threatens 'reductionism' or a dominating agenda (and even a return to eugenics) fails to address the enormous expansion of knowledge and its impact for good as well as for ill on contemporary society. The idea that such disciplines are only 'one way of understanding reality', discursive 'fabrications' or, worse, merely ideological edifices, underestimates the issues at stake and detracts from serious analysis.

Medical sociology needs the confidence to reject superficial critiques of – let alone outright hostility to – 'biology' and 'biomedicine', and instead to provide a detailed and critical appreciation of their development and inter-relationship. If the body is to be invoked in sociological enquiry, and especially in medical sociology, then the place of the biological sciences (as well as the biological dimensions of experience) have to be more clearly appreciated. Sociological analysis needs to incorporate their impact on lay experience and the assimilation of the knowledge they produce about the body by lay populations (the healthy, the sick and the disabled), especially as it is mediated through social movements and the mass media. Certainly the development of the 'new genetics' is bringing us into a new relationship with what the nineteenth-century French physician Claud Bernard called the *milieu intérieur* of the body.

The new genetics is also highlighting the links between the body and risk. Today questions are being posed about the limits of what counts as 'the body' and how these limits are being redrawn. The phenomenological, social and ethical dimensions of these new forms of knowledge all need to be taken more seriously by medical sociology than they have been to date. Certainly the impact of genetic testing on professional and lay people's views of chronic illness and disability is likely to provide potentially new areas of debate. There are signs, however, that medical sociologists are now making a positive contribution to understanding in this area (Davison *et al.* 1994; Richards 1993; Marteau and Richards 1996). Empirical work which is developing on lay views of risk and genetics and how far these differ from professional views (e.g. Parsons and Atkinson 1992) could benefit in the future from making clearer links with the body. As scientific knowledge gathers speed, one of the most important questions in this respect will be how lay people manage to assimilate statistical information and produce new forms of lay knowledge about bodily processes which will inform their actions.

Even the most cursory reading of popular writing in the biological sciences today, for example that of the British geneticist Steve Jones (1993, 1996), indicates the enormous power of the explanatory models being employed and the extent of the manipulation of the natural world, including the body, to which they relate. If medical sociology wishes to come to terms with 'corporeal realities' it will also have to come to terms (as does sociology as a whole) with the limits of its own explanatory powers, and the relationship between its own frames of reference and those of other disciplines, including the biological and medical sciences. The lack of confidence that is expressed in avoiding these issues, for fear of biological determinism, reductionism and the like, can only reduce the discipline's impact. It has been the argument throughout this book that in addressing health, illness and the impact of the bio-medicine in a changing society, medical sociology can continue to contribute to mainstream sociological thought. More importantly, in engaging with such issues medical sociology can help to address some of the most important personal and social problems of the twenty-first century.

References

Able Smith, B. and Townsend, P. (1965) *The Poor and the Poorest*, London: Bell & Son.

Albrecht, G. (1992) *The Disability Business*, London: Sage.

Album, D. (1989) 'Patients' knowledge and patients' work: patient–patient interaction in general hospitals', *Acta Sociologica* 32, 3: 295–306.

Alderson, M. (1988) 'Demographic and health trends in the elderly', in N. Wells and C. Freer (eds) *The Ageing Population: Burden or Challenge?* Houndsmills, Basingstoke: Macmillan.

Andrews, A. and Jewson, N. (1993) 'Ethnicity and infant deaths: the implications of recent statistical evidence for materialist explanations', *Sociology of Health and Illness* 15, 2: 137–156.

Arber, S. (1990) 'Opening the black box: inequalities in women's health', in P. Abbott and G. Payne (eds) *New Directions in the Sociology of Health*, Basingstoke: Falmer Press.

——(1994) 'Gender, health and ageing', *Medical Sociology News* 20, 1: 14–22.

Arber, S. and Evandrou, M. (eds) (1993) *Ageing, Independence and the Life Course*, London: Jessica Kingsley Publishers.

Arber, S. and Ginn, J. (1991) *Gender and Later Life: A Sociological Analysis of Resources and Constraints*, London: Sage.

Arie, T. (1988) Foreword, in N. Wells and C. Freer (eds) *The Ageing Population: Burden or Challenge?* Houndsmills, Basingstoke: Macmillan.

Ariès, P. (1981) *The Hour of Our Death*, London: Allen Lane.

Arksey, H. (1994) 'Expert and lay participation in the construction of medical knowledge', *Sociology of Health and Illness* 16, 4: 448–468.

Armstrong, D. (1987) 'Silence and truth in death and dying', *Social Science and Medicine* 24: 651–657.

——(1993) 'Public health spaces and the fabrication of identity', *Sociology* 27, 3: 393–410.

——(1995) 'The rise of surveillance medicine', *Sociology of Health and Illness* 17, 3: 393–440.

Audit Commission (1993) *What Seems to be the Matter: Communication Between Hospitals and Patients*, London: HMSO.

Backett, K.C. and Davison, C. (1995) 'Lifecourse and lifestyle: the social and cultural location of health behaviours', *Social Science and Medicine* 40, 5: 629–638.

Balarajan, R. and Bulusu, L. (1990) 'Mortality among immigrants in England and Wales, 1979–1983', in M. Britton (ed.) *Mortality and Geography: A Review in the Mid 1980s*, OPCS series DS No. 9, London: HMSO.

Baldwin, S. and Falkingham, J. (eds) (1994) *Social Security and Social Change: New Challenges to the Beveridge Model*, Hemel Hempstead: Harvester Wheatsheaf.

Barnes, C. (1991) *Disabled People in Britain and Discrimination*, London: Hurst & Co.

Barnes, C. and Oliver, M. (1995) 'Disability rights: rhetoric and reality in the UK', *Disability and Society* 10, 1: 111–116.

Barrett, M. and Roberts, H. (1978) 'Doctors and their patients: the social control of women in general practice', in C. Smart and B. Smart (eds) *Women, Sexuality and Social Control*, London: Routledge and Kegan Paul.

Bartley, M. (1994) 'Unemployment and ill health: understanding the relationship', *Journal of Epidemiology and Community Health* 48: 333–337.

Baudrillard, J. (1993) *Symbolic Exchange and Death*, London: Sage.

Bauman, Z. (1989) *Modernity and the Holocaust*, Cambridge: Polity Press.

——(1992) *Mortality, Immortality and Other Life Strategies*, Cambridge: Polity Press.

——(1994) 'Morality without ethics', *Theory Culture and Society* 11: 1–34.

Beck, U. (1992) *Risk Society: Towards a New Modernity*, London: Sage.

Bendelow, G. and Williams, S. (1994) 'Review. Emotions and the body: raising the issues for medical sociology', *Medical Sociology News* 19, 2: 38–44.

——(1995) 'Transcending the dualisms: towards a sociology of pain', *Sociology of Health and Illness* 17, 2: 139–165.

Benton, T. (1991) 'Biology and social science: why the return of the repressed should be given a (cautious) welcome', *Sociology* 25, 1: 1–29.

Benzeval, M., Judge, K. and Whitehead, M. (eds) (1995) *Tackling Inequalities in Health: An Agenda for Action*, London: King's Fund.

Berger, P. and Kellner, H. (1981) *Sociology Reinterpreted*, Harmondsworth: Penguin Books.

Berger, P. and Luckmann, T. (1967) *The Social Construction of Reality: A Treatise in the Sociology of Knowledge*, London: Allen Lane.

Berger, P., Berger, B. and Kellner, H. (1974) *The Homeless Mind*, Harmondsworth: Penguin Books.

Berkman, L.F. and Breslow, L. (1983) *Health and Ways of Living: the Almeda County Study*, Oxford: Oxford University Press.

Berridge, V. and Strong, P. (1991) 'AIDS and the relevance of history', *Social History of Medicine* 4, 1: 129–138.

Black, D. (1994) *A Doctor Looks at Health Economics*, London: Office of Health Economics.

Blane, D., Davey Smith, G. and Bartley, M. (1993) 'Social selection: what does it contribute to social class differences in health?', *Sociology of Health and Illness* 15: 2–15.

Blaxter, M. (1976) *The Meaning of Disability*, London: Heinemann.

——(1983) 'The causes of disease: women talking', *Social Science and Medicine* 17: 59–69.

——(1990) *Health and Lifestyles*, London: Routledge.

——(1992) 'Inequality in health and the problem of time', *Medical Sociology News* 18, 1: 12–24.

——(1993) 'Why do the victims blame themselves', in A. Radley (ed.) *Worlds of Illness: Biographical and Cultural Perspectives on Health and Disease*, London: Routledge.

Blaxter, M. and Paterson, E. (1982) *Mothers and Daughters*, London: Heinemann.

Bloor, M. (1976) 'Professional autonomy and client exclusion: a study of ENT clinics', in M. Wadsworth and D. Robinson (eds) *Studies in Everyday Medical Life*, Oxford: Martin Robertson.

——(1995a) *The Sociology of HIV Transmission*, London: Sage.

——(1995b) 'A user's guide to contrasting theories of HIV-related risk behaviour', in J. Gabe (ed.) *Medicine, Health and Risk: Sociological Approaches*, Oxford: Blackwell.

Bloor, M. and Horobin, G. (1975) 'Conflict and conflict resolution in doctor–patient relationships', in C. Cox and A. Mead (eds) *A Sociology of Medical Practice*, London: Collier Macmillan.

Bloor, M. and McIntosh, J. (1990) 'Surveillance and concealment: a comparison of client resistance in therapeutic communities and health visiting', in S. Cunningham-Burley and N. McKeganey (eds) *Readings in Medical Sociology*, London: Tavistock/Routledge.

Blumer, H. (1971) 'Social problems as collective behaviour', *Social Problems* 18, 3: 298–306.

Bowling, A. (1991) *Measuring Health*, Buckingham: Open University Press.

——(1995) *Measuring Disease*, Buckingham: Open University Press.

Brindle, D. (1995) 'Survey charts increasing gulf between top earners and poor', *Guardian*, 26 January.

British Medical Journal (1986) 'Lies, damned lies and suppressed statistics' (editorial) 293: 349–350.

Brown, J. C. (1994) 'Poverty in post-war Britain', in J. Obelkevich and P. Catterall (eds) *Understanding Post-War British Society*, London: Routledge.

Brown, P. (1995) 'Popular epidemiology, toxic waste and social movements', in J. Gabe (ed.) *Medicine, Risk and Health*, Oxford: Blackwell.

Bruce, I., McKennel, A. and Walker, E. (1991) *Blind and Partially Sighted People in Great Britain*, London: HMSO.

Burns, T. (1992) *Erving Goffman*, London: Routledge.

Burrows, R. and Loader, B. (eds) (1994) *Towards a Postfordist Welfare State?* London: Routledge.

Burrows, R. and Nettleton, S. (1995) 'Going against the grain: smoking and "heavy" drinking amongst the British middle classes', *Sociology of Health and Illness* 17, 5: 668–680.

Bury, M. (1979) 'Disability in society: towards an integrated perspective', *International Journal of Rehabilitation Research* 2, 1: 33–40.

——(1982) 'Chronic illness as biographical disruption', *Sociology of Health and Illness* 4, 2: 167–182.

——(1986) 'Social constructionism and the development of medical sociology', *Sociology of Health and Illness* 8, 2: 137–169.

——(1987) 'The international classification of impairments, disabilities and handicaps: a review of research and prospects', *International Disability Studies* 9, 3: 118–122.

——(1988) 'Arguments about ageing: long life and its consequences', in N. Wells and C. Freer (eds) *The Ageing Population: Burden or Challenge?* Houndsmills, Basingstoke: Macmillan.

——(1991) 'The sociology of chronic illness: a review of research and prospects', *Sociology of Health and Illness* 13, 4: 451–468.

——(1992a) 'The future of ageing: changing perceptions and realities', in J.C. Brockelhurst, R.C. Tallis and H. Fillit (eds) *Textbook of Geriatric Medicine and Gerontology* (4th edn) London: Churchill Livingstone.

——(1992b) 'Medical sociology and chronic illness: a comment on the panel discussion', *Medical Sociology News* 18, 1: 29–33.

——(1994a) 'Quality of life: why now? A sociological view', in L. Nordenfelt (ed.) *Concepts and Measurement of Quality of Life in Health Care*, Dordrecht: Kluwer.

——(1994b) 'Health promotion and lay epidemiology: a sociological view', *Health Care Analysis* 2: 23–30.

——(1994c) 'Health and and chronic illness: a sociological view', *Health Care Analysis* 2, 3: 240–246.

——(1996a) 'Defining and researching disability: challenges and responses', in C. Barnes and G. Mercer (eds) *Exploring the Divide: Illness and Disability*, Leeds: The Disability Press.

——(1996b) 'Disability and the myth of the independent researcher', *Disability and Society* 11, 1: 111–113.

Bury, M. and Gabe, J. (1994) 'Television and medicine: medical dominance or trial by media', in J. Gabe, D. Kelleher and G. Williams (eds) *Challenging Medicine*, London: Routledge.

Busfield, J. (1994) 'The female malady? Men, women and madness in 19th century Britain', *Sociology* 28: 259–277.

Bynum, W.F. (1994) *Science and the Practice of Medicine in the Nineteenth Century*, Cambridge: Cambridge University Press.

Calnan, M. (1987) *Health and Illness: the Lay Perspective*, London: Tavistock.

——(1994) ' "Lifestyle" and its social meaning', in G. Albrecht (ed.) *Advances in Medical Sociology* vol. 4, Greenwich, Conn.: JAI Press.

Calnan, M. and Gabe, J. (1991) 'Recent developments in General Practice', in J. Gabe, M. Calnan and M. Bury (eds) *The Sociology of the Health Service*, London: Routledge.

Calnan, M. and Johnson, B. (1985) ' Health, health risks and inequalities: an exploratory study of women's perceptions', *Sociology of Health and Illness* 7: 55–75.

Campbell, J. and Oliver, M. (1996) *Disability Politics: Understanding Our Past, Changing Our Future*, London: Routledge.

Cant, S. and Calnan, M. (1991) 'On the margins of the medical market place: an exploratory study of alternative practitioners' perceptions', *Sociology of Health and Illness* 13, 1: 39–57.

Carr-Hill, R. (1992) 'The measurement of patient satisfaction', *Journal of Public Health Medicine* 14, 3: 236–249.

Carricaburu, D. and Pierret, J. (1995) 'From biographical disruption to biographical reinforcement: the case of HIV-positive men', *Sociology of Health and Illness* 17, 1: 65–88.

Cartwright, A. (1967) *Patients and Their Doctors*, London: Routledge and Kegan Paul.

Cartwright, A. and Anderson, R. (1981) *General Practice Revisited: A Second Study of Patients and Their Doctors*, London: Tavistock.

Cartwright, A. and O'Brien, M. (1976) 'Social class variations in health care and the nature of general practitioner consultations', in M. Stacey (ed.) *The Sociology of the NHS*, Sociological Review Monograph No. 22, Keele: University of Keele.

Cartwright, A., Hockey, L. and Anderson, J.L. (1973) *Life before Death*, London: Routledge and Kegan Paul.

Central Statistical Office (CSO) (1995) *Social Trends 25*, London: HMSO.

Clarke, K., Gray, D., Keeting, N.A. and Hampton, J.R. (1994) 'Do women with acute myocardial infarction receive the same treatment as men?' *British Medical Journal* 309: 563–566.

Cochrane, A. (1972) *Effectiveness and Efficiency: Random Reflections on the Health Service*, London: Nuffield Provincial Hospital Trust.

Comaroff, J. (1982) 'Medicine, symbol and ideology', in P. Wright and A. Treacher (eds) *The Problem of Medical Knowledge: Examining the Social Construction of Medicine*, Edinburgh: Edinburgh University Press.

Comaroff, J. and Maguire, P. (1981) 'Ambiguity and the search for meaning: childhood leukaemia in the modern clinical context', *Social Science and Medicine* 15B: 115–123.

Conover, P. (1973) 'Social class and chronic illness', *International Journal of Health Services* 3, 3: 357–368.

Conrad, P. (1992) 'Medicalisation and social control', *Annual Review of Sociology* 18: 209–232.

——(1994) 'Wellness as virtue: morality and the pursuit of health', *Culture, Medicine and Psychiatry* 18: 385–401.

Corbin, J. and Strauss, A. (1988) *Unending Work and Care: Managing Chronic Illness at Home*, San Francisco: Jossey-Bass.

——(1991) 'Comeback: the process of overcoming disability', in G.L. Albrecht and J.A. Levy (eds) *Advances in Medical Sociology* vol. 2, Greenwich, Conn.: JAI Press.

Cornwell, J. (1984) *Hard-Earned Lives: Accounts of Health and Illness From East London*, London: Tavistock.

Cottingham, J. (1986) *Descartes*, Oxford: Blackwell.

Coward, R. (1989) *The Whole Truth: The Myth of Alternative Health*, London: Faber and Faber.

Crawford, R. (1977) 'You are dangerous to your health: the ideology and politics of victim blaming', *International Journal of Health Services* 7: 663–680.

Crawford, R. (1980) 'Healthism and the medicalization of everyday life', *International Journal of Health Services* 19: 365–388.

——(1984) 'A cultural account of "health": control, release and the social body', in K. McKinlay (ed.) *Issues in the Political Economy of Health Care*, London: Tavistock.

Davey, B. (1996) 'Personal experiences, professional explanations', in B. Davey and C. Seale (eds) *Experiencing and Explaining Disease*, Buckingham: Open University Press.

Davey Smith, G., Bartley, M. and Blane, D. (1990) 'The Black Report on socio-economic inequalities in health ten years on', *British Medical Journal* 310: 373–377.

——(1991) 'Black on class and health: a reply to Strong', *Journal of Public Health Medicine* 13: 350–357.

Davey Smith, G., Blane, D. and Bartley, M. (1994) 'Explanations for socio-economic differentials in mortality: evidence from Britain and elsewhere', *European Journal of Public Health* 4: 131–144.

Davison, C., Davey Smith, G. and Frankel, S. (1991) 'Lay epidemiology and the prevention paradox: the implications of coronary candidacy for health promotion', *Sociology of Health and Illness* 13, 1: 1–19.

Davison, C., Frankel, S. and Davey Smith, G. (1992) 'The limits of popular lifestyle: re-assessing "fatalism" in the popular culture of illness prevention', *Social Science and Medicine* 34, 6: 675–685.

Davison, C., Macintyre, S. and Davey Smith, G. (1994) 'The potential social impact of predictive genetic testing for susceptibility to common chronic diseases: a review and proposed research agenda', *Sociology of Health and Illness* 16, 3: 340–371.

Department of Health (1991) *The Patient's Charter*, London: HMSO.

Department of Health and Social Security (1976) *Prevention and Health: Everybody's Business*, London: HMSO.

de Vauss, D.A. (1990) *Surveys in Social Research* (2nd edn) London: Unwin Hyman.

Dingwall, R. (1976) *Aspects of Illness*, London: Martin Robertson.

Dingwall, R., Fenn, P. and Quam, L. (1991) *Medical Negligence: a Review and Bibliography*, Oxford: Centre for Socio-Legal Studies, Wolfson College.

Donovan, J.L., Frankel, S.J. and Eyles, J.D. (1993) 'Assessing the need for health status measures', *Journal of Epidemiology and Community Health* 47: 158–162.

Douglas, M. (1966) *Purity and Danger: An Analysis of the Concepts of Pollution and Taboo*, London: Routledge and Kegan Paul.

——(1973) *Natural Symbols: Explorations in Cosmology*, Harmondsworth: Penguin Books.

Doyal, L. (1994) 'Changing medicine? Gender and the politics of health care', in J. Gabe, D. Kelleher and G. Williams (eds) *Challenging Medicine*, London: Routledge.

———(1996) *What Makes Women Sick*, London: Macmillan.

Dubos, R. (1960) *Mirage of Health*, London: Allen and Unwin.

Eisenberg, L. (1977) 'Disease and illness: distinctions between popular and professional ideas of sickness', *Culture, Medicine and Psychiatry*, 1: 9–23.

Elias, N. (1978) *The History of Manners: The Civilizing Process* vol. 1, Oxford: Blackwell.

———(1982) *State Formation and Civilization: The Civilizing Process* vol. 2, Oxford: Blackwell.

———(1985) *The Loneliness of the Dying*, Oxford: Blackwell.

Elston, M. A. (1991) 'The politics of professional power: medicine in a changing health service', in J. Gabe, M. Calnan and M. Bury (eds) *The Sociology of the Health Service*, London: Routledge.

Engel, G.L. (1977) 'The need for a new medical model: a challenge for bio-medicine', *Science* 196: 129–136.

Epstein, R.A. (1976) 'Medical malpractice: the case for contract', *American Bar Foundation Research Journal* 76: 87–149.

———(1977) 'Contracting out of the medical malpractice crisis', *Perspectives in Biology and Medicine* 20: 228–245.

Ettorre, E. and Riska, E. (1995) *Gendered Moods: Psychotropics and Society*, London: Routledge.

Evans, R. (1987) *Death in Hamburg: Society and Politics in the Cholera Years, 1830–1910*, Oxford: Oxford University Press.

Fagerhaugh, S. (1975) 'Getting round with emphysema', in A. Strauss (ed.) *Chronic Illness and the Quality of Life*, St Louis: Mosby.

Featherstone, M. (1991) *Consumer Culture and Postmodernism*, London: Sage.

Featherstone, M. and Hepworth, M. (1991) 'The mask of ageing and the postmodern life course', in M. Featherstone, M. Hepworth and B.S. Turner (eds) *The Body: Social Processes and Cultural Theory*, London: Sage.

Field, D. (1989) *Nursing the Dying*, London: Tavistock/Routledge.

Field, D. and James, N. (1993) 'Where and how people die', in D. Clark (ed.) *The Future for Palliative Care: Issues of Policy and Practice*, Buckingham: Open University Press.

Finklestein, V. (1980) *Attitudes and Disabled People: Issues for Discussion*, New York: World Rehabilitation Fund.

Fitzpatrick, R. and Albrecht, G. (1994) 'The plausibility of quality of life measures in different domains of health care', in L. Nordenfelt (ed.) *Concepts and Measurement of Quality of Life in Health Care*, Dordrecht: Kluwer.

Fitzpatrick, R., Bury, M. and Donnelly, T. (1987) 'Problems in the assessment of outcome in a back pain clinic', *International Disability Studies* 9: 161–165.

Fitzpatrick, R., McLean, J., Boulton, M., Hart, G. and Dawson, J. (1989) 'Variation in sexual behaviour in gay men', in *AIDS: Social Representations and Social Practices*, Basingstoke: Falmer Press.

Foster, P. (1989) 'Improving the doctor–patient relationship', *Journal of Social Policy* 18, 3: 337–361.

Fox, A.J., Goldblatt, P.O. and Jones, D.R. (1986) 'Social class mortality differentials: artefact, selection or life circumstances?', in R.G. Wilkinson (ed.) *Class and Health: Research and Longitudinal Data*, London: Tavistock.

Fox, N.J. (1993) *Postmodernism, Sociology and Health*, Buckingham: Open University Press.

Freidson, E. (1970a [and 1988]) *Profession of Medicine: A Study of the Sociology of Applied Knowledge*, Chicago: University of Chicago Press.

——(1970b) *Professional Dominance*, New York: Atherton.

——(1989) *Medical Work in America: Essays on Health Care*, Yale: Yale University Press.

French, S. (1993) 'Disability, impairment or something in between?', in J. Swain, V. Finkelstein, S. French and M. Oliver (eds) *Disabling Barriers – Enabling Environments*, London: Sage.

Gabe, J. (1995) 'Health, medicine and risk: the need for a sociological approach', in J. Gabe (ed.) *Medicine, Health and Risk: Sociological Approaches*, Oxford: Blackwell.

Gabe, J. and Bury, M. (1996) 'Risking tranquilliser use: cultural and lay dimensions', in S.J. Williams and M. Calnan (eds) *Modern Medicine: Lay Perspectives and Experiences*, London: UCL Press.

Gabe, J. and Thorogood, N. (1986) 'Prescribed drugs and the management of everyday life: the experience of black and white working-class women', *Sociological Review* 34: 737–772.

Gabe, J., Calnan, M. and Bury, M. (eds) (1991) Introduction to *The Sociology of the Health Service*, London: Routledge.

Gabe, J., Kelleher, D. and Williams, G. (eds) (1994) *Challenging Medicine*, London: Routledge.

Gallagher, E. (1976) 'Lines of reconstruction and extension in the Parsonian sociology of illness', *Social Science and Medicine* 10: 207–218.

Gellner, E. (1992) *Postmodernism, Reason and Religion*, London: Routledge.

Gerhardt, U. (1979) 'The Parsonian paradigm and the identity of medical sociology', *Sociological Review* 27: 229–251.

——(1987) 'Parsons, role theory and health interaction', in G. Scambler (ed.) *Sociological Theory and Medical Sociology*, London: Tavistock.

——(1989) *Ideas About Illness: An Intellectual and Political History of Medical Sociology*, London: Macmillan.

——(1990) 'Introductory essay: qualitative research in chronic illness: the issue and the story', *Social Science and Medicine* 30: 1149–1159.

Giddens, A. (1989) *Sociology*, Cambridge: Polity Press.

——(1991) *Modernity and Self Identity*, Cambridge: Polity Press.

——(1994) *Beyond Left and Right: the Future of Radical Politics*, Cambridge: Polity Press.

Glaser, B. and Strauss, A. (1964) 'Awareness contexts and social interaction', *American Sociological Review* 29: 669–679.

——(1965) *Awareness of Dying*, Chicago: Aldine.

——(1967) *The Discovery of Grounded Theory*, Chicago: Aldine.

Goffman, E. (1971) *The Presentation of Self in Everyday Life*, Harmondsworth: Penguin Books.

Goldthorpe, J.H., Llewellyn, C. and Payne, C. (1980) *Social Mobility and Class Structure in Modern Britain*, Oxford: Oxford University Press.

Good, Byron J. (1994) *Medicine, Rationality and Experience: An Anthropological Perspective*, Cambridge: Cambridge University Press.

Gordon, G. (1966) *Role Theory and Illness: A Sociological Perspective*, New Haven: College and University Press.

Graham, H. (1987) 'Women's smoking and family health', *Social Science and Medicine* 25, 1: 47–56.

——(1993) *When Life's a Drag: Women, Smoking and Disadvantage*, London: HMSO.

Green, D. (ed.) (1988) *Acceptable Inequalities? Essays on the Pursuit of Equality*, London: Institute of Economic Affairs.

Gregory, S. and Hartley, G.M. (eds) (1991) *Constructing Deafness*, London: Pinter Publishers in association with the Open University.

Grosz, E. (1994) *Volatile Bodies: Towards a Corporeal Feminism*, Bloomington and Indianapolis: Indiana University Press

Hammersley, M. (1992) 'On feminist methodology', *Sociology* 26, 2: 187–206.

Hannay, D.R. (1979) *The Symptom Iceberg: A Study of Community Health*, London: Routledge and Kegan Paul.

Hannington, W. (1937) *The Problem of the Distressed Areas*, London: Gollancz.

Harré, R. (1991) *Physical Being: A Theory for a Corporeal Psychology*, Oxford: Blackwell.

Harris, A., Cox, E. and Smith, C. (1970) *Handicapped and Impaired in Great Britain* vol. 1, London: HMSO.

——(1971) *Handicapped and Impaired in Great Britain, Economic Dimensions*, London: HMSO.

Harwood, R.H., Rogers, A., Dickinson, E. and Ebrahim, S. (1994) 'Measuring handicap: the London handicap scale, a new outcome measure for chronic disease', *Quality in Health Care* 3: 11–16.

Hassan, I. (1985) 'The culture of postmodernism', *Theory Culture and Society* 2, 3: 119–131.

Healy, B. (1991) 'The Yentl syndrome', *New England Journal of Medicine* 325: 272–277.

Helman, C. (1981) ' "Tonic", "fuel" and "food": social and symbolic aspects of the long-term use of psychotropic drugs', *Social Science and Medicine* 15B: 521–533.

Hennessy, P. (1996) *Muddling Through; Power, Politics and the Quality of Government in Post-War Britain*, London: Gollancz.

Herzlich, C. (1973) *Health and Illness: A Social Psychological Analysis*, London: Academic Press.

Hirst, P. and Woolley, P. (1982) *Social Relations and Human Attributes*, London: Tavistock.

Hockey, J. (1986) 'The human encounter with death: an anthropological approach', Ph.D. thesis, University of Durham.

Hollingshead, A.B. and Redlich F.C. (1958) *Social Class and Mental Illness*, New York: John Wiley and Sons.

Holton, R.J. and Turner, B.S. (eds) (1986) *Talcott Parsons on Economy and Society*, London: Routledge.

Hunter, D.J. (1994) 'From tribalism to corporatism: the managerial challenge to medical dominance', in J. Gabe, D. Kelleher and G. Williams (eds) *Challenging Medicine*, London: Routledge.

Illich, I. (1975) *Medical Nemesis*, London: Calder and Boyars.

Illsley, R. (1980) *Professional or Public Health? Sociology in Health and Medicine*, London: Nuffield Provincial Hospitals Trust.

——(1986) 'Occupational class, selection and the production of inequalities in health', *Quarterly Journal of Social Affairs* 2: 151–165.

——(1987) 'The health divide, bad welfare or bad statistics?', *Poverty* 67: 16–17.

Illsley, R. and Baker, D. (1991) 'Contextual variations in the meaning of health inequality', *Social Science and Medicine* 32: 359–365.

Illsley, R. and Le Grand, J. (1987) 'The measurement of inequality in health', in A. Williams (ed.) *Economics and Health*, London: Macmillan.

Jefferys, M. (1986) 'The transition from public health to community medicine: the evolution and execution of a policy for occupational transformation', *Bulletin of the Society for the Social History of Medicine* 39: 47–63.

——(1991) 'Medical sociology and public health', *Public Health* 105: 15–21.

Jefferys, M. and Sachs, H. (1983) *Rethinking General Practice*, London: Tavistock.

Jefferys, M. and Thane, P. (1989) 'Introduction: an ageing society and ageing people', in M. Jefferys (ed.) *Growing Old in the Twentieth Century*, London: Routledge.

Jefferys, M., Nullard, J.B., Hyman, M. and Warren, M.D. (1969) 'A set of tests for measuring motor impairment in prevalence studies', *Journal of Chronic Diseases* 28: 303–309.

Jennett, B. (1988) 'The elderly and high technology therapies', in N. Wells and C. Freer (eds) *The Ageing Population: Burden or Challenge?* Houndsmills, Basingstoke: Macmillan.

Jobling, R. (1988) 'The experience of psoriasis under treatment', in R. Anderson and M. Bury (eds) *Living with Chronic Illness: The Experience of Patients and Their Families*, London: Unwin Hyman.

Jones, S. (1993) *The Language of the Genes*, London: Flamingo.

——(1996) *In the Blood: God, Genes and Destiny*, London: HarperCollins.

Judge, K. (1995) 'Income distribution and life expectancy: a critical appraisal', *British Medical Journal* 311: 1282–1285.

Kadushin, C. (1966) 'Social class and the experience of health', in R. Bendix and S.M. Lipset (eds) *Class Status and Power*, New York: Free Press.

Kane, R.L., Klein, S.J., Bernstein, L. *et al.* (1985) 'Hospice role in alleviating the emotional stress of terminal patients and their families', *Medical Care* 23: 189–197.

Karpf, A. (1988) *Doctoring the Box*, London: Routledge.

Kellehear, A. (1984) 'Are we a death-denying society? A sociological review', *Social Science and Medicine* 18, 9: 713–723.

——(1990) *Dying of Cancer: The Final Year of Life*, Chur and London: Harwood Academic Publishers.

Kelleher, D. (1988) *Diabetes*, London: Routledge.

Kelly, M. (1992) *Colitis*, London: Routledge.

——(1995) 'Narrative analysis and chronic illness', inaugural lecture, University of Greenwich.

Kelly, M. and Field, D. (1994) 'Comments on the rejection of the bio-medical model in sociological discourse', *Medical Sociology News* 19, 3: 34–37.

——(1996) 'Medical sociology, chronic illness and the body', *Sociology of Health and Illness* 18, 2: 241–257.

Klein, R. (1988) 'Acceptable inequalities', in D. Green (ed.) *Acceptable Inequalities? Essays on the Pursuit of Equality*, London: Institute of Economic Affairs.

——(1991) 'Making sense of inequalities: a response to Peter Townsend', *International Journal of Health Services* 21, 1: 175–181.

Kleinman, A. (1988) *The Illness Narratives: Suffering, Healing and the Human Condition*, New York: Basic Books.

Kronenfeld, J.J. and Glik, D.C. (1991) 'Perceptions of risk: its applicability in medical sociological research', *Research in the Sociology of Health Care* 9: 307–344.

Kubler Ross, E. (1970) *On Death and Dying*, London: Tavistock.

Lasch, C. (1979) *The Culture of Narcissism*, London: Sphere Books.

Lash, S. and Urry, J. (1987) *The End of Organised Capitalism*, Cambridge: Polity Press.

Law, C.M. (1994) 'Employment and industrial sector', in J. Obelkevich and P. Catterall (eds) *Understanding Post-War British Society*, London: Routledge.

Lawrence, C. (1995) *Medicine in the Making of Modern Britain 1700–1920*, London: Routledge.

Lazarus, R.S. (1985) 'The costs and benefits of denial', in A. Monat and R. S. Lazarus (eds) *Stress and Coping: An Anthology* (2nd edn), New York: Columbia University Press.

Lee, R. (1993) *Doing Research on Sensitive Topics*, London: Sage.

Lenny, J. (1993) 'Do disabled people need counselling?', in J. Swain, V. Finkelstein, S. French and M. Oliver (eds) *Disabling Barriers – Enabling Environments*, Milton Keynes: Open University Press.

Long, A. (1994) 'Assessing health and social outcomes', in J. Popay and G. Williams (eds) *Researching the People's Health*, London: Routledge.

Lupton, D. (1994) *Medicine as Culture*, London: Sage.

——(1995) *The Imperative of Health: Public Health and the Regulated Body*, London: Sage.

Lyotard, J.-F. (1984) *The Postmodern Condition: A Report on Knowledge*, Manchester: Manchester University Press.

Macdonald, L. (1988) 'The experience of stigma: living with rectal cancer', in R. Anderson and M. Bury (eds) *Living with Chronic Illness: The Experience of Patients and Their Families*, London: Unwin Hyman.

McIntosh, J. (1977) *Communication and Awareness in a Cancer Ward*, London: Croom Helm.

Macintyre, S. (1986) 'The patterning of health by social position in contemporary Britain: directions for sociological research', *Social Science and Medicine* 23, 4: 393–415.

——(1994) 'Understanding the social patterning of health: the role of the social sciences', *Journal of Public Health Medicine* 16, 1: 53–59.

McKeown, T. (1976) *The Role of Medicine: Dream, Mirage or Nemesis?*, London: Nuffield Provincial Hospitals Trust.

McKinlay, J. B. (1973) 'Social networks, lay consultation and help-seeking behaviour', *Social Forces* 51: 279–292.

Magee, B. (1987) *The Great Philosophers*, London: BBC Books.

Manning, P. and Fabrega, H. (1973) 'The experience of self and body: health and illness in the Chiapas Highlands'; in G. Psathas (ed.) *Phenomenological Sociology*, New York: Wiley.

Marmot, M., Adelstein, A. and Bulusu, L. (1984) *Immigrant Mortality in England and Wales: 1970–1978*, OPCS Studies on Population and Medical Subjects No. 47, London: HMSO.

Marsh, C. (1982) *The Survey Method: the Contribution of Surveys to Sociological Explanation*, London: Allen and Unwin.

Marteau, T. and Richards, M. (1996) *The Troubled Helix: Social and Psychological Implications of the New Genetics*, Cambridge: Cambridge University Press.

Martin, B. (1981) *A Sociology of Contemporary Cultural Change*, Oxford: Blackwell.

——(1991) 'The cultural construction of ageing: or how long can the summer wine really last?', in M. Bury and J. Macnicol (eds) *Aspects of Ageing: Essays in Social Policy and Old Age*, Egham: Department of Social Policy and Social Science, Royal Holloway.

Martin, E. (1987) *The Woman in the Body*, Milton Keynes: Open University Press.

——(1990) 'The end of the body?', *American Ethnologist*: 121–139.

Martin, J., Meltzer, H. and Elliott, D. (1988) *The Prevalence of Disability Among Adults*, London: HMSO.

Mechanic, D. (1968 [2nd edn 1978]) *Medical Sociology: A Selective View*, New York: Free Press.

Mellor, P. (1993) 'Death in high modernity: the contemporary presence and absence of death', in D. Clark (ed.) *The Sociology of Death*, Oxford: Blackwell.

Mills, C. Wright (1959) *The Sociological Imagination*, Harmondsworth: Penguin Books.

Mishler, E.G. (1984) *The Discourse of Medicine: Dialectics of Medical Interviews*, New Jersey: Ablex Publishing Co.

Mohan, J. (1991) 'Privatization in the British health sector: a challenge to the NHS?', in J. Gabe, M. Calnan and M. Bury (eds) *The Sociology of the Health Service*, London: Routledge.

——(1996) *A National Health Service? The Restructuring of Health Care in Britain Since 1979*, London: Macmillan.

Morgan, J. (1988) 'Living with renal failure on home dialysis', in R. Anderson and M. Bury (eds) *Living with Chronic Illness: The Experience of Patients and Their Families*, London: Unwin Hyman.

Morgan, M. (1989) 'Social ties, support and well-being', in D. Patrick and H. Peach (eds) *Disablement in the Community*, Oxford: Oxford Medical Publications.

——(1996) 'The meaning of high blood pressure among Afro-Caribbean and white patients', in D. Kelleher and S. Hillier (eds) *Researching Cultural Differences in Health*, London: Routledge.

Mouzelis, N.P. (1991) *Back to Sociological Theory*, Basingstoke: Macmillan.

Mulkay, M. (1993) 'Social death in Britain', in D. Clark (ed.) *The Sociology of Death*, Oxford: Blackwell.

Murphy, R. (1994) 'The sociological construction of science without nature', *Sociology* 28, 4: 957–974.

Nettleton, S. (1995) *The Sociology of Health and Illness*, Cambridge: Polity Press.

Nettleton, S. and Harding, G. (1994) 'Protesting patients: a study of complaints made to a family health service authority', *Sociology of Health and Illness* 16, 1: 38–61.

Nietzsche, F. (1969) *Thus Spoke Zarathustra*, Harmondsworth: Penguin Books.

——(1979) *Ecce Homo*, Harmondsworth: Penguin Books.

Nordenfelt, L. (1993) *Quality of Life, Health and Happiness*, Aldershot: Avebury.

Oakley, A. (1980) *Women Confined: Towards a Sociology of Childbirth*, Oxford: Martin Robertson.

——(1984) *The Captured Womb: A History of the Medical Care of Pregnant Women*, Oxford: Blackwell.

——(1992) *Social Support and Motherhood*, Oxford: Blackwell.

Obelkevich, J. and Catterall, P. (eds) (1994) *Understanding Post-War British Society*, London: Routledge.

Oliver, M. (1990) *The Politics of Disablement*, London: Macmillan.

——(1992) 'Changing the social relations of research production', *Disability, Handicap and Society* 7, 2: 101–114.

——(1996) *Understanding Disability: From Theory to Practice*, London: Macmillan.

Oliver, M., Zarb, G., Silver, J., Moore, M. and Salisbury, V. (1988) *Walking into Darkness: The Experience of Spinal Injury*, London: Macmillan.

Ots, T. (1990) 'The angry liver, the anxious heart and the melancholy spleen: the phenomenology of perceptions in Chinese culture', *Culture, Medicine and Psychiatry* 14: 21–58.

Parsons, E. and Atkinson, P. (1992) 'Lay constructions of genetic risk', *Sociology of Health and Illness* 14: 437–455.

Parsons, T. (1951) *The Social System*, New York: Free Press.

——(1958) 'Health and illness in the light of American values and social structure', in E.G. Jaco (ed.) *Patients, Physicians and Illness*, New York: Free Press.

——(1978) 'The sick role and the role of the physician reconsidered', in *Action Theory and the Human Condition*, New York: Free Press.

Parsons, T. and Fox, R. (1952) 'Illness, therapy and the modern American family', *Journal of Social Issues* 8: 31–44.

Patrick, D. (1986) 'Evaluating health care', in D. Patrick and G. Scambler (eds) *Sociology as Applied to Medicine*, London: Ballière Tindall.

Patrick, D. and Peach, H. (eds) (1989) *Disablement in the Community*, Oxford: Oxford Medical Publications.

Perakyla, A. (1989) 'Appealing to the "experience" of the patient in the care of the dying', *Sociology of Health and Illness* 11, 2: 117–134.

Petticrew, M., McKee, M. and Jones, J. (1993) 'Coronary artery surgery: are women discriminated against?', *British Medical Journal* 306: 1164–1166.

Pill, R. and Stott, N.C.H. (1982) 'Concepts of illness causation and responsibility: some preliminary data from a sample of working-class mothers', *Social Science and Medicine* 16: 43–52.

——(1985) 'Preventive procedures and practices among working-class women: new data and fresh insights', *Social Science and Medicine* 21: 975–993.

Pill, R., Peters, T.J. and Robling, M.R. (1993) 'Factors associated with health behaviour among mothers of lower socio-economic status: a British example', *Social Science and Medicine* 36, 9: 1137–1144.

Pinder, R. (1995) 'Bringing back the body without the blame? The experience of ill and disabled people at work', *Sociology of Health and Illness* 17, 5: 605–631.

Polhemus, T. (ed.) (1978) *Social Aspects of the Human Body*, Harmondsworth: Penguin Books.

Pope, C. and Mays, N. (1995) 'Qualitative research: reaching the parts other methods cannot reach: an introduction to qualitative methods in health and health services research', *British Medical Journal* 311: 42–45.

Popper, K., Lindahl, B.I.B. and Arhem, P. (1993) 'A discussion of the mind brain problem', *Theoretical Medicine* 14: 167–180.

Porter, M. (1990) 'Professional–client relationships and women's reproductive health care', in S. Cunningham-Burley and N. McKeganey (eds) *Readings in Medical Sociology*, London: Tavistock/Routledge.

Pound, P., Bury, M., Gompertz, P. and Ebrahim, S. (1995) 'Stroke patients' views on their admission to hospital', *British Medical Journal* 311: 18–22.

Powles, J. (1972) 'On the limitations of modern medicine', *Science, Medicine and Man* 1, 1: 1–30.

Radley, A. (1994) *Making Sense of Illness*, London: Sage.

Rayner, G. and Stimson, G. (1979) 'Medicine, superstructure and micropolitics – a response', *Social Science and Medicine* 13A: 611–612.

Richards, M.P.M. (1993) 'The new genetics: some issues for social scientists', *Sociology of Health and Illness* 15, 5: 567–586.

Riessman, C.K. (1993) *Narrative Analysis*, London: Sage.

Riley, M.W., Foner, A. and Waring, J. (1988) 'Sociology of age', in N.J. Smelser (ed.) *Handbook of Sociology*, London and Newbury Park: Sage.

Roberts, H. (1985) *Women : The Patient Patients*, London: Pandora Press.

Roberts, R., Brunnner, E., White, I. and Marmot, M. (1993) 'Gender differences in occupational mobility and structure of employment in the British civil service', *Social Science and Medicine* 37, 12: 1415–1425.

Robinson, D. (1971) *The Process of Becoming Ill*, London: Routledge and Kegan Paul.

——(1973) *Patients, Practitioners and Medical Care*, London: Heinemann.

Robinson, I. (1988) *Multiple Sclerosis*, London: Routledge.

Rose, G. (1985) 'Sick individuals and sick populations', *International Journal of Epidemiology* 14: 32–38.

Roth, J.A. (1963) *Timetables: Structuring the Passage of Time in Hospital Treatment and Other Careers*, Indianapolis: Bobbs Merrill.

Runciman, W.G. (1966) *Relative Deprivation and Social Justice: A Study of Attitudes to Social Inequality in Twentieth-Century England*, London: Routledge and Kegan Paul.

Saks, M. (ed.) (1992) *Alternative Medicine in Britain*, Oxford: Clarendon Press.

Samson, C. (1995) in *Independent on Sunday*, 20 August 1995.

Scambler, A., Scambler, G. and Craig, D. (1981) 'Kinship and friendship networks and women's demand for primary care', *Journal of the Royal College of General Practitioners* 26: 746–750.

Scambler, G. and Hopkins, A. (1988) 'Accommodating epilepsy in families', in R. Anderson and M. Bury (eds) *Living with Chronic Illness: The Experience of Patients and Their Families*, London: Unwin Hyman.

Scheff, T. (1966) *Being Mentally Ill: A Sociological Theory*, Chicago: Aldine.

Scheper-Hughes, N. and Lock, M.M. (1987) 'The mindful body: a prolegomenon to future work in medical anthropology', *Medical Anthropology Quarterly* 1: 6–41.

Schneider, J.W. and Conrad, P. (1983) *Having Epilepsy: The Experience and Control of Epilepsy*, Philadelphia: Temple University Press.

Seale, C. (1989) 'What happens in hospices: a review of research evidence', *Social Science and Medicine* 28, 6: 551–559.

——(1995) 'Society and death', in B. Davey (ed.) *Birth to Old Age: Health in Transition*, Buckingham: Open University Press.

Seale, C. and Cartwright, A. (1994) *The Year Before Death*, Aldershot: Avebury.

Sen, A. (1984) 'Poor, relatively speaking', in A. Sen (ed.) *Resources, Values and Development*, Oxford: Blackwell.

Shakespeare, T. (1993) 'Disabled people's self organisation: a new social movement', *Disability and Society* 8, 3: 249–264.

Sharma, U. (1992) *Complementary Medicine Today: Practitioners and Patients*, London: Routledge.

Shilling, C. (1993) *The Body and Social Theory*, London: Sage.
Shoemaker, S. (1984) *Identity, Cause and Mind*, Cambridge: Cambridge University Press.
Silverman, D. (1987) *Communication and Medical Practice: Social Relations in the Clinic*, London: Sage.
Singer, E. (1974) 'Premature social ageing: the social psychological consequences of a chronic illness', *Social Science and Medicine* 8: 143–151.
Smaje, C. (1995) *Health, 'Race' and Ethnicity: Making Sense of the Evidence*, London: King's Fund Institute.
Small, N. (1993 'Dying in a public space: AIDS deaths', in D. Clark (ed.) *The Sociology of Death*, Oxford: Blackwell.
Social Science and Medicine (1994) 'Special issue: narrative representations of illness and healing', *Social Science and Medicine* 38, 6.
Stacey, M. (1976) 'The health service consumer: a sociological misconception', in *The Sociology of the NHS*, Sociological Review Monograph No. 22, Keele: University of Keele.
——(1988) *The Sociology of Health and Healing*, London: Unwin Hyman.
Stacey, M. and Homans, H. (1978) 'The sociology of health and illness: its present state, future prospects and potential for health research', *Sociology* 12: 281–307.
Standing Medical Advisory Committee (1994) *Management of Lung Cancer: Current Clinical Practices*, London: HMSO.
Stern, J. (1983) 'Social mobility and the interpretation of social class mortality differentials', *Journal of Social Policy* 12: 27–49.
Stimson, G. (1974) 'Obeying doctor's orders: a view from the other side', *Social Science and Medicine* 8: 97–104.
——(1976) 'General practitioners: trouble and types of patients', in M. Stacey (ed.) *The Sociology of the NHS*, Sociological Review Monograph No. 22, Keele: University of Keele.
Stimson, G. and Webb, B. (1975) *Going to See the Doctor: the Consultation Process in General Practice*, London: Routledge and Kegan Paul.
Stone, D.A. (1984) *The Disabled State*, London: Macmillan.
Strauss, A. (ed.) (1975) *Chronic Illness and the Quality of Life*, St Louis: Mosby.
Strauss, A. and Corbin, J. (1988) *Shaping a New Health Care System: The Exploration of Chronic Illness As a Catalyst for Change*, San Francisco: Jossey Bass.
Strauss, A., Fagerhaugh, S., Suczek, B. and Wiener, C. (1982) 'Sentimental work in the technological hospital', *Sociology of Health and Illness* 4: 254–278.
Strauss, A., Schatzman, L., Ehrlich, D., Bucher, R. and Sabshin, M. (1963) 'The hospital and its negotiated order', in E. Freidson (ed.) *The Hospital and Modern Society*, London: Free Press.
Strong, P. (1979a) 'Sociological imperialism and the profession of medicine', *Social Science and Medicine* 13A: 199–215.
——(1979b) *The Ceremonial Order of the Clinic: Parents, Doctors and Medical Bureaucracies*, London: Routledge and Kegan Paul.
——(1979c) 'Materialism and medical interaction: a critique of "medicine,

superstructure and micropolitics"', *Social Science and Medicine* 13A: 613–619.

——(1990a) 'Black on class and mortality; theory, method and history', *Journal of Public Health Medicine* 12: 168–180.

——(1990b) 'Epidemic psychology: a model', *Sociology of Health and Illness* 12, 3: 249–259.

Sudnow, D. (1967) *Passing On: The Social Organization of Dying*, Englewood Cliff, NJ: Prentice Hall.

Szasz, T. and Hollander, M. (1956) 'A contribution to the philosophy of medicine: the basic models of the doctor–patient relationship', *Archives of Internal Medicine* 97: 589–592.

Szreter, S. (1988) 'The importance of social interaction in Britain's mortality decline – 1850–1914: a re-interpretation of the role of public health', *Bulletin of the Society for the Social History of Medicine* 41:1–37.

Taylor, C. (1989) *Sources of the Self: The Making of the Modern Identity*, Cambridge: Cambridge University Press.

——(1991) *The Ethics of Authenticity*, Cambridge, Mass.: Harvard University Press.

Taylor, D. (1977) *Physical Impairment: Social Handicap*, London: Office of Health Economics.

Taylor, R.C.R. (1984) 'Alternative medicine and the medical encounter in Britain and the United States', in J. Warren Salmon (ed.) *Alternative Medicines: Popular and Policy Perspectives*, London: Tavistock.

Timmermans, S. (1994) 'Dying of awareness: the theory of awareness contexts revisited', *Sociology of Health and Illness*, 16, 3: 322–339.

Topliss, E. (1979) *Provision for the Disabled* (2nd edn), Oxford: Blackwell with Martin Robertson.

Totman, R. (1990) *Mind, Stress and Health*, London: Souvenir Press.

Townsend, P. (1979) *Poverty in the United Kingdom*, Harmondsworth: Penguin Books.

——(1981) 'The structured dependency of the elderly: a creation of social policy in the twentieth century', *Ageing and Society* 1, 1: 5–28.

——(1990) 'Widening inequalities of health in Britain: a rejoinder to Rudolph Klein', *International Journal of Health Services* 20, 3: 363–370.

——(1991) 'Evading the issue of widening inequalities of health in Britain: a reply to Rudolf Klein', *International Journal of Health Services* 21, 1: 183–189.

Townsend, P. and Davidson, N. (1982, Penguin edition 1990) *Inequalities in Health: The Black Report*, Harmondsworth: Penguin Books.

Tuckett, D., Boulton, M., Olson, C. and Williams, A. (1985) *Meetings Between Experts*, London: Tavistock.

Turner, B. (1984) *The Body and Society: Explorations in Social Theory*, Oxford: Blackwell.

——(1992) *Regulating Bodies: Essays in Medical Sociology*, London: Routledge.

Turner, V. (1974) *The Ritual Process*, Harmondsworth: Penguin Books.

Vagero, D. (1995) 'Health inequalities as policy issues – reflections on

ethics, policy and public health', *Sociology of Health and Illness* 17, 1: 1–19.
Vagero, D. and Illsley, R. (1995) 'Explaining health inequalities: beyond Black and Barker', *European Sociological Review* 11, 3: 219–241.
Wadsworth, M., Butterfield, W.J.H. and Blaney, R. (1971) *Health and Sickness: The Choice of Treatment*, London: Tavistock.
Waitzkin, H. (1979) 'Medicine, superstructure and micropolitics', *Social Science and Medicine* 13A: 601–609.
——(1984) 'The micropolitics of medicine: a contextual analysis', *International Journal of Health Services* 14, 3: 339–377.
Walker, A. (1981) 'Towards a political economy of old age', *Ageing and Society* 1, 1: 73–94.
Walter, T. (1991) 'The mourning after Hillsborough', *Sociological Review* 39, 3: 599–625.
——(1994) *The Revival of Death*, London: Routledge.
Watney, S. (1987) *Policing Desire: Pornography, AIDS and the Media*, London: Comedia.
Webster, C. (1994) 'Tuberculosis', in C. Seale and S. Pattison (eds) *Medical Knowledge: Doubt and Certainty*, Buckingham: Open University Press.
Wedderburn, D. (1965) 'Facts and theories of the welfare state', in R. Miliband (ed.) *The Socialist Register*, London: Merlin Press.
Wells, N. (1984) 'Changing patterns of disease', in J. Teeling Smith (ed.) *A New NHS Act for 1996?*, London: Office of Health Economics.
Westergaard, T. and Resler, H. (1976) *Class in a Capitalist Society*, Harmondsworth: Penguin Books.
Whitehead, M. (1990, revised 1992) *The Health Divide*, Harmondsworth: Penguin Books.
Wiener, C. (1975) 'The burden of rheumatoid arthritis: tolerating the uncertainty', *Social Science and Medicine* 9: 97–104.
Wilkinson, R. (1986) 'Income and mortality', in R. Wilkinson (ed.) *Class and Health*, London: Tavistock.
——(1992) 'Income distribution and life expectancy', *British Medical Journal* 304: 165–168.
——(1994) 'Health redistribution and growth', in A. Glynn and D. Miliband (eds) *Paying for Inequality: the Economic Costs of Social Injustice*, London: Rivers Oram Press.
——(1996) *Unhealthy Societies: From Inequality to Well-Being*, London: Routledge.
Williams, G. (1984) 'The genesis of chronic illness: narrative reconstruction', *Sociology of Health and Illness* 6: 175–200.
Williams, G. and Popay, J. (1994) 'Lay knowledge and the privilege of experience', in J. Gabe, D. Kelleher and G. Williams (eds) *Challenging Medicine*, London: Routledge.
Williams, G., Fitzpatrick, R., MacGregor, A. and Rigby, A.S. (1996) 'Rheumatoid arthritis', in B. Davey and C. Seale (eds) *Experiencing and Explaining Disease*, Buckingham: Open University Press.
Williams, R. (1990) *A Protestant Legacy: Attitudes to Death and Illness Among Older Aberdonians*, Oxford: Clarendon Press.

——(1993) 'The health costs of Britain's industrialisation', in S. Platt, H. Thomas, S. Scott and G. Williams (eds) *Locating Health: Sociological and Historical Explorations*, Aldershot: Avebury.

——(1994) 'Medical, economic and population factors in areas of high mortality: the case of Glasgow', *Sociology of Health and Illness* 16, 2: 143–181.

Williams, S.J. (1993) *Chronic Respiratory Disorder*, London: Routledge.

Williams, S.J. and Bendelow, G. (1996) 'Emotions, health and illness: the "missing link" in medical sociology?', in V. James and J. Gabe (eds) *Health and the Sociology of Emotions*, Oxford: Blackwell.

Williams, S.J. and Bury, M. (1989) 'Impairment, disability and handicap in chronic respiratory illness', *Social Science and Medicine* 29, 5: 609–616.

Witz, A. (1994) 'The challenge of nursing', in J. Gabe, D. Kelleher and G. Williams (eds) *Challenging Medicine*, London: Routledge.

World Health Organisation (1980) *International Classification of Impairments, Disabilities and Handicaps*, Geneva: WHO.

Wyke, S. and Ford, G. (1992) 'Competing explanations for associations between marital status and health', *Social Science and Medicine* 34, 5: 523–532.

Young, A. (1980) 'The discourse on stress and the reproduction of conventional knowledge', *Social Science and Medicine* 14B: 133–146.

Young, A. (1981) 'When Rational Man falls sick: an inquiry into some assumptions made by medical anthropologists', *Cultural Medicine and Psychiatry* 5: 317–335.

Young, E., Bury, M. and Elston, M.A. (1994) 'Emotions apart: some methodological issues in prospective work with dying women', paper given at BSA Medical Sociology Conference, University of York.

Young, M. and Cullen, L. (1996) *A Good Death: Conversations with East Londoners*, London: Routledge.

Zola, I. (1972) 'Medicine as an institution of social control', *Sociological Review* 20: 487–504.

——(1973) 'Pathways to the doctor – from person to patient', *Social Science and Medicine* 7: 677–89.

Index